D0423081

Psychological Abuse
in Violent
Domestic Relations

K. Daniel O'Leary, PhD, is Distinguished Professor of Psychology and past Chairman of the Psychology Department of the State University of New York at Stony Brook. He is a clinical psychologist who received his doctoral degree from the University of Illinois at Urbana, Illinois in 1967. Dr. O'Leary was among the top 100 psychologists in the English-speaking world, as cited by the *American Psychologist* in December 1978. He received the Distinguished Scientist Award from the clinical division (12, Section III) of the American Psychological Association in 1985, and was installed to the National Academies of Practice in Psychology in 1986. He is a Fellow of the American Psychological Association (Divisions 7, 12, and 25), and was president of the American Association for Advancement of Behavior Therapy. Dr. O'Leary is the author or coauthor of nine books, including: *Marital Therapy Treatment for Depression* (1990), *Abnormal Psychology* (1996), and *The Couples Psychotherapy Treatment Planner* (1998). His research focuses on the etiology and treatment of partner aggression, and the marital discord/depression link.

Roland D. Maiuro, PhD, is the Director of the Anger Management, Domestic Violence, and Workplace Conflict Programs located at Harborview Medical Center in Seattle, and Associate Professor in the Department of Psychiatry and Behavioral Sciences at the University of Washington School of Medicine. He was a Henry Rutgers Scholar at Rutgers University, and earned his doctoral degree in clinical psychology at Washington University in St. Louis. Dr. Maiuro has received the Social Issues Award from the Washington State Psychological Association for his research on domestically violent men, and the Gold Achievement Award from the American Psychological Association for program development, teaching, and applied research in the areas of anger and interpersonal violence. Dr. Maiuro currently serves as Editor-in-Chief for *Violence and Victims*, an internationally distributed research journal devoted to theory, practice, and public policy related to perpetrators and victims of interpersonal violence.

Psychological Abuse in Violent Domestic Relations

K. Daniel O'Leary, PhD
and Roland D. Maiuro, PhD

Editors

 Springer Publishing Company

Copyright © 2001 by Springer Publishing Company, Inc.

Springer Publishing Company, Inc.
536 Broadway
New York, NY 10012-3955

Cover design by Susan Hauley
Cover photograph by Bernhard Springer
Acquisitions Editor: Bill Tucker
Production Editor: Elizabeth Keech

01 02 03 04 05 / 5 4 3 2 1

Library of Congress Cataloging-in-Publication Data

Psychological abuse in violent domestic relations / K. Daniel O'Leary and Roland D. Maiuro, editors.

    p.   cm.
A compilation of articles from the journal Violence and Victims
Includes bibliographical references and index.
ISBN 0-8261-1321-4 (hardcover)
1. Family violence—Psychological aspects. 2. Psychological abuse. I. O'Leary, K. Daniel, 1940- II. Maiuro, Roland D.

RC569.5.F3 P787 2000
616.85'822—dc21
                                          99-059298

Printed in Canada by Trigraphic Printing

Contents

Contributors

Courtney Ahrens, PhD
Department of Psychology
University of Illinois
Chicago, IL

Ileana Arias, PhD
Department of Psychology
The University of Georgia
Athens, GA

Lauren Bennett, PhD
Department of Psychology
University of Maryland
Baltimore, MD

Amy Blickenstaff, PhD
Department of Psychology
University of Illinois
Chicago, IL

Doris Williams Campbell, ARNP, PhD
College of Nursing
University of South Florida
Tampa, FL

Jacquelyn Campbell, PhD, RN, FAAN
School of Nursing
Johns Hopkins University
Baltimore, MD

Mary Ann Dutton, PhD
George Washington University
Law Center
Bethesda, MD

Mary Farrington, PhD
Department of Psychology
University of Cincinnati
Cincinnati, OH

Janet Foliano, PhD
Department of Psychology
University of Cincinnati
Cincinnati, OH

Lisa A. Goodman, PhD
Department of Psychology
University of Maryland
Baltimore, MD

Dee L. R. Graham, PhD
Department of Psychology
University of Cincinnati
Cincinnati, OH

Rachel Hacker, PhD
Department of Psychology
University of Cincinnati
Cincinnati, OH

Sherry L. Hamby, PhD
Family Research Laboratory
University of New Hampshire
Durham, NH

Sharon A. Hoover, PhD
Department of Psychology
University of Maryland
Baltimore, MD

Kim Ihms, PhD
Department of Psychology
University of Cincinnati
Cincinnati, OH

Christine King
School of Nursing
University of Massachusetts
Amherst, MA

Diane Latimer, PhD
Department of Psychology
University of Cincinnati
Cincinnati, OH

Linda L. Marshall, PhD
Department of Psychology
University of North Texas
Denton, TX

Christopher M. Murphy, PhD
Department of Psychology
University of Maryland
Baltimore, MD

Karen T. Pape, PhD
Department of Psychology
The University of Georgia
Athens, GA

Barbara Parker, PhD, RN, FAAN
School of Nursing
University of Virginia
Charlottesville, VA

Edna I. Rawlings, PhD
Department of Psychology
University of Cincinnati
Cincinnati, OH

Stephanie Riger, PhD
Department of Psychology
University of Illinois
Chicago, IL

Josephine Ryan, PhD, RN
School of Nursing
University of Massachusetts
Amherst, MA

Leslie A. Sackett, PhD
Columbia College
Columbia, SC

Daniel G. Saunders, PhD
University of Michigan
School of Social Work
Ann Arbor, MI

Kelly Suttman, PhD
Department of Psychology
University of Cincinnati
Cincinnati, OH

Alicia Thompson, PhD
Department of Psychology
University of Cincinnati
Cincinnati, OH

Richard M. Tolman, PhD
University of Michigan
School of Social Work
Ann Arbor, MI

Preface

Sticks and Stones May Break My Bones, But Names Will Also Hurt Me: Psychological Abuse in Domestically Violent Relationships

E arly studies of domestic violence among intimate partners were based on sociological and criminological theory. As a result, the early focus was upon behavioral acts, which often constituted a transgression of acceptable cultural norms or a violation of another person's rights in the form of indexed criminal behavior. However, as the field has evolved, other disciplines have joined in the study of domestic violence including clinical psychology, social work, nursing, and, more recently, emergency and primary care medicine. As a result, domestic violence is now viewed as a cluster or pattern of interrelated behaviors, which can not only impact another person's freedom and rights but also effect various aspects of physical health and emotional well-being. A comprehensive definition of domestic violence now includes all behaviors that exert physical force to injure, control, or abuse an intimate or family member, forced or coerced sexual activity, destruction of property, acts which threaten or abuse family pets, as well as nonphysical acts that threaten, terrorize, personally denigrate, or restrict freedom (Rosenbaum & Maiuro, 1989).

DIMENSIONS OF PSYCHOLOGICAL ABUSE

Critical review of the current literature on domestic violence and abuse reveals that the terminology used to describe psychological and emotional abuse varies from writer to writer. Terms such as psychological abuse, psychological maltreatment, verbal abuse, mental abuse, emotional abuse or maltreatment, and "psychological violence" are commonly used interchangeably. While some writers use these terms synonymously to refer to nonphysical forms of abuse, others may make distinctions between them. Psychological and emotional abuse, which may include behaviors such as name-calling, verbal yelling, coercive and controlling tactics either in the presence or absence of physical abuse, are sometimes differentiated from "psychological violence" which occurs only in association with physical violence, thereby carrying an implied threat of physical violence and the associated power to intimidate or control another person. For the purposes of the present volume, the terms psychological and emotional abuse are used interchangeably. However, for purposes of conceptual clarity and scientific rigor, the terms *violence* or *battery* will be used in their more traditional sense and restricted to actual physical acts of abuse.

Table 1 provides a summary of four primary dimensions of psychological abuse among intimate partners and examples of each type of abuse for introductory and descriptive purposes. Given the endless number of tactics that could conceivably be used to psychologically aggress against an intimate partner, psychologically abusive behaviors are organized according to areas of impact upon the victim. As will be observed in the papers included in this text, there are a variety of ways of conceptualizing and defining psychological abuse. These conceptual frames include the action or intent of the perpetrator, the emotional impact upon the victim, or the area of life-functioning that is affected. The "best" classification schema (i.e., that which is most explanatory, predictive, or useful in terms of intervention) has yet to be determined. The actual theoretical or practical utility of conceptualizing and classifying various types of psychological abuse will be determined by empirical studies. One of the aims of the present text is to provide a solid foundation for this work.

As one examines the state of the current paradigm for the study of psychological abuse, a number of questions come to the fore. Some of these follow: Can psychological abuse be defined and described? Can it be measured? Does it have meaningful relationships with other forms of abuse? Does it explain unique variance related to traumatic impact upon victims? As reflected in the

TABLE 1. Dimensions of Psychological Abuse in Domestically Violent Relationships

---

I. Denigrating Damage to Partner's Self-Image or Esteem

Yelling; referring to partner in profane, derogatory and demeaning terms; name calling; put-downs regarding appearance and behavior; shaming or embarrassing in front of friends and family; attempts to disaffect or alienate children; being hyper-critical; negativism; ridiculing, invalidating feelings; projecting personal responsibility through blame; focusing upon the person rather than his/her behavior.

II. Passive-Aggressive Withholding of Emotional Support and Nurturance

---

Punitive use of avoidance and withdrawal, sulking, silent treatment, spiteful inaction, neglect, emotional abandonment.

III. Threatening Behavior: Explicit and Implicit

Threats to physically hurt, disfigure, or kill; coercive threats to divorce, to take away the children; lying and infidelity; engaging in reckless driving or behavior.

IV. Restricting Personal Territory and Freedom

Isolation from friends and family; stalking or checking on whereabouts; invading diary or telephone records; preventing partner from working or going to school or doing things on their own; dominating decision making with the relationship; controlling partner's money; exit blocking; interfering with partner's use of telephone; taking car keys or disabling the car; sex-role stereotyping, (i.e., "a woman's place is..."); controlling partner's options on the basis of gender and/or marital status, a sense of entitlement or ownership.

---

contents of this volume, important progress has been made with regard to all of these questions. The purpose of this book is to provide an overview of new developments in theory, research, and practice related to psychological abuse in domestically violent relationships. As much of this work has previously appeared in the peer-reviewed journal *Violence and Victims*, it reflects some of the current state of the art and science of our understanding. It is hoped that the present compilation and integration of this work will provide an accessible resource for researchers, practitioners, and policy makers concerned with evolving and expanding our efforts to end all forms of domestic violence and abuse.

MEASUREMENT ISSUES

O'Leary critically reviews the status of psychological abuse as a "variable deserving critical attention." This attention is deemed critical due to the relative neglect of psychological abuse in comparison to physical abuse. It is asserted that not only does psychological abuse attend most forms of physical abuse but that it is also deleterious to health and well-being in its own right. Indeed, in victimization studies which have included interview and measurement protocols for emotional abuse, it is often the psychological aspects of abuse which are cited as most devastating to a relationship (cf. Follingstad, Rutledge, Berg, Hause, & Polek, 1990). A recent study of 1,152 women recruited from family practice clinics indicated that women experiencing psychological abuse were likely to report physical health problems such as arthritis, chronic pain, migraine, sexually transmitted disease, and stomach ulcers, even when the effect of physical violence is removed or adjusted in the data (Coker, Smith, Bethee, King, & McKeown, 2000). Moreover, research data have begun to accumulate which suggests that psychological abuse may precede physical abuse during the course of some relationships (Leonard & Senchak, 1996; Murphy & O'Leary, 1989; O'Leary, Malone, & Tyree, 1994). In addition, there is preliminary evidence to support the notion that, as in the case of physical abuse, children exposed to recurrent witnessing of psychological abuse such as yelling may have lasting sequelae in the form of increased risk for anxiety, depression, and interpersonal problems (Blumenthal, Neeman, & Murphy, 1998).

As the quality of research in any area is only as good as the measurement tools available to investigate it, O'Leary also provides an overview of available measures of psychological abuse. He concludes that the construct can now be reliably measured. O'Leary's review of these scales should provide readers with useful information for selecting a measure appropriate for their research focus or clinical practice.

Murphy and Hoover explore the feasibility and utility of assessing psychological abuse as a multifactorial construct. Based on a systematic review of the literature on emotional abuse in marital and dating relationships (Murphy & Cascardi, in press), a four-factor model is proposed. These factors include Hostile Withdrawal, Domination/Intimidation, Denigration, and Restrictive Engulfment. A provisional 54-item measure incorporating these four factors is then tested on two samples of college-aged women in dating relationships.

The authors report data to support the construct validating the proposed four-factor model of psychological abuse. Moreover, preliminary data are analyzed to suggest that two forms of psychological abuse, Dominance/Intimidation and Denigration, may be more closely related to physical violence than either Hostile Withdrawal or Restrictive Engulfment. It should be noted that dehumanizing forms of labeling have occurred in most major wars due to their power to facilitate aggression and allow the enemy to be attacked without remorse. The identification of the types of psychological abuse that precede physical violence may have important utility for premarital counseling efforts. In this sense they may be helpful for identifying at-risk couples and modifying dysfunctional conflict resolution strategies before they evolve to the point of physical violence.

Since its initial publication in *Violence and Victims* in 1989, Tolman's psychological maltreatment of women inventory has been an important tool for advancing our empirical understanding of psychological abuse in domestically violent relationships. In the present volume, Tolman provides further data on the validity of the measure using the "known groups" method of determining criterion validity, as well as studies of convergent and discriminant validity. As the reader will observe, questions still remain regarding our ability to assess severity of impact and a reliable cutting score to determine, on a pure psychometric basis, who is psychologically abused and who is not.

Of all constructs, male dominance is perhaps the one most closely associated with feminist theories of domestic violence (Coleman & Straus, 1986; Koss et al., 1994). Drawing upon a new conceptualization of dominance (Hamby, Poindexter, & Gray-Little, 1996), Hamby provides data related to the development of a dominance scale with a convenience sample of 131 undergraduate students. Of theoretical interest is the author's attempt to differentiate between authoritarian dominance, in which one partner exercises more decision-making power than the other, and restrictive dominance, in which one partner feels entitled and exercises the "right" to violate or intrude upon the other partner's behavior and decision-making in areas of life that do not otherwise involve them (e.g., choice of friends, personal activities). The study results suggest that authoritarian dominance relates only to psychological aggression while restrictive dominance is positively correlated with both psychological and physical aggression as well as injury. Hamby additionally observes that it is impossible to determine whether an individual's scores reflect a unilateral attempt to dominate or a reciprocal response to either a power struggle or some form of abuse. It is suggested that couple data may be necessary to assess dyadic interplay such as the relative use of power and control tactics.

Some theoretical and clinical investigators have compared the psychological abuse that transpires in domestic partner relationships to a form of terrorism (cf. Lenore Walker [1994] for a discussion of the Amnesty International definition of terrorism as it applies to domestic violence). Graham and colleagues take the line of thinking an important step forward, with their development of a scale for identifying the "Stockholm Syndrome" in victimized women. As previously described by Graham and colleagues (1994), this syndrome conceptualizes the domestic violence victim as a "hostage" kept captive by the "traumatic bond" (cf. Dutton & Painter, 1993) established with the perpetrator. In its fully developed state, victims deny both their terror and abuse and identify with the perceived "kind side" of their aggressive captor.

Graham's scale is of both theoretical and clinical interest in that it assesses the impact or outcome of various types of psychological abuse including a) threat to survival, b) an addictive conditioning to the variable, partial, and unpredictable kind side of the abuser, c) isolation from friends and family and other support who might offer an alternative perspective, d) lack of personal freedom to escape or avoid punishment outside of placating the more powerful abuser. This syndrome also offers an alternative explanation to some of the existing simplistic theories of why many women stay in abusive relationships (e.g., fear and economics) and appear "resistant" to attempts to assist them. It also offers an interesting alternative to PTSD models of victim trauma that may not fully capture the special circumstances and dynamics of battered woman's syndrome. Moreover, as a psychometric instrument, it has the advantage of being able to assess the features of the syndrome on a continuum as opposed to a dichotomous diagnostic, presence or absence basis.

It is often pointed out that domestic violence and abuse cuts across all racial, ethnic, and socioeconomic strata. Despite the common underscoring of this fact at many education venues and in the text of many fact sheets on the topic, precious little has been done to ensure the use of culturally sensitive instruments, protocols and assessments. In a special issue of *Violence and Victims* devoted to violence against women of color, important data were reported relating to the incidence of marital abuse, child abuse, harassment, and accessibility of Hispanic, African American, and Native American populations. After conducting a national survey of 142 partner abuse programs, Williams and Becker (1994) reported that little or no effort has been made to understand or accommodate the special needs of minority populations.

Given this context, Campbell and colleagues' empirical study of the reliability and factor structure of the Index of Spouse Abuse with an African American population represents a particularly important addition to this text. The Hudson and McIntosh (1981) measure represents one of the first attempts to evaluate psychological abuse in the context of ongoing physical abuse. The work by Campbell and colleagues reveals a somewhat different and more differentiated factor structure than that originally reported by Hudson and McIntosh. Consistent with other studies, there appears to be both a verbal aggressive aspect as well as a controlling and isolating dimension. Importantly, the study provides support for the use of the ISA with African American women, while at the same time it provides psychometric support for a cautious and culturally sensitive interpretation of findings in light of interpersonal and psychological dynamics documented for this ethnic group. It also provides a good example of the type of carefully conducted work that is needed to operationalize the concept of cultural competency in our assessment protocols for domestic violence.

INTERRELATIONSHIPS AND OUTCOMES

For psychological abuse to be fully grounded as a scientific construct, it must have more than descriptive properties. It must show meaningful relationships within victim trauma or the course or progression of perpetrator and/or victim behavior. Arias and Pape examine the relationship of psychological abuse to both PTSD symptoms and intention to leave an abusive partner. The investigators found a more complex relationship between decisions to leave and PTSD symptoms than would be predicted by simply looking at levels of physical and psychological abuse. This study has clear implications for understanding the psychological well-being of battered women and our ability to offer assistance, which is attuned to both their emotional and situational vulnerability and circumstance. The authors use of "ways of coping" as a moderating variable in the analysis of their data also helps integrate an understanding of battered women in the context of methodology employed in stress and coping research.

Given the heavy reliance upon the criminal justice system as a means of protecting battered women, it is surprising that there have not been more studies of the relationship between types of abuse and women's help-seeking through the courts. Dutton, Goodman, and Bennett provide data on women seeking various combinations of civil protection orders and criminal prosecution against a perpetrator. The role of various types of psychological, physical, and sexual abuse was studied to evaluate their impact alone and in combination. As with previous studies, modest albeit significant correlations, were found between these measures supporting the notion that psychological abuse is a separate but identifiable aspect of the abuse experience. Importantly, the continued centrality of physical abuse as a predictor of battered women's willingness to engage the legal system as well as leave a domestic relationship was underscored by their work. In contrast, the relatively stronger role of psychological abuse in producing traumatic response in the form of depression and PTSD symptoms was also supported. Their work underscores the value of viewing domestic violence from an interdisciplinary perspective whereby traumatic outcomes can be defined in terms of criminological, physical health, and mental health effects.

In keeping with the prior observations that psychological abuse may have many themes and variations in terms of tactics employed, Marshall provides a rich and different perspective drawn from social psychological and communication theories. Based on her earlier studies demonstrating that psychological abuse may be quite subtle in nature and veiled in pseudo-loving or quasi-humorous tones (Marshall, 1994, 1996), Marshall examines both obvious or overt as well as more subtle forms of psychological abuse. The author concludes that the more subtle forms of abuse are likely to be used more frequently and have a cumulative, debilitating impact upon the victim's "sense of self," fear, perceived relationship quality, and general quality of life. Less support was found for dominating and controlling forms of abuse despite the frequency of its being cited in the current literature as the central form and dynamic of men's abuse against women. Although the study sample is limited to low-income women, the sensitivity and multifaceted quality of Marshall's assessment protocol provides a fine example of a sophisticated approach to the phenomena of psychological abuse.

Sackett and Saunders further extend our understanding of psychological abuse by examining the relative impact of various types of psychological abuse upon both sheltered and non-sheltered female victims. Factor analytic procedures are employed that differentiate four major forms of abuse including criticizing behavior, ridiculing personal traits, jealous control, and ignoring. Evidence is found to support the notion that critical attacks upon a victim's personality or personal traits may have more severe impact than critical attacks upon their behavior. The finding that jealous and controlling forms of psychological abuse were closely related to physical abuse is also important. Specifically, it suggests that meaningful relationships may exist between psychological and physical forms of abuse that may provide tools for identifying potential victims of physical violence at earlier stages of abuse or in the absence of frank admissions of violence that may be withheld by victims due to fear of reprisal.

CONCLUDING COMMENTARY

The present work reflects significant advances in our ability to assess and understand psychological abuse in domestically violent relationships. However, we are far from developing reliable "norms" regarding these behaviors. As Tolman observes, there is no cutting score that reliably determines when someone reaches the point of being psychologically abused.

As with any clinically meaningful and scientific construct, it is important that a definition be developed that is not overinclusive. In this regard, psychological abuse cannot simply be "all about power and control" when the question can be rhetorically asked…What isn't? As human beings we all strive for self-empowerment, personal self-efficacy, and internal locus of control. In fact, such characteristics have been associated with positive self-esteem and good health as opposed to pathology and dysfunction. Efforts such as Hamby's preliminary effort at refining and differentiating the critical construct of dominance into "authority" and "restrictiveness" dimensions helps lend important insight into the type of boundary violations that constitute the abusive use of power and control.

Another possible direction is to develop an assessment approach, which not only assesses the presence and frequency of psychological abuse but also subjective impact. While O'Leary's recommendation that we develop a standard akin to physical abuse which minimally requires at least two instances of domestic abuse to establish a recurrent pattern or one that is severe enough to require medical attention has some merit, there may also be qualitative as a well as quantitative differences in certain types of behavior that gives them the potential to do harm. For example, proponents of the concept of "psychological battery" or "psychological violence" make the point that certain acts of psychological abuse (e.g., threats to harm) become more powerful in the context of a history of physical abuse than they would be in isolation by virtue of their ability to revivify actual violence through post-traumatic processes. Whether the distinction offered between psychological violence and psychological abuse is purely arbitrary or descriptive in nature, the fact remains that such a distinction is an attempt to begin to differentiate the concept of psychological abuse in domestically violent relationships from dysfunctional communications observed in the context of marital discord (Burman, Margolin, & John, 1993). For the paradigm to evolve further in this area, there will be a need for research designs which include appropriate control and comparison groups and statistical analyses to ferret out substantive differences in levels of abuse. An example of such a design is a three-way analysis with domestically violent, maritally discordant but not violent, and maritally satisfied and nonviolent participants.

The need to develop more sophisticated assessment techniques is further underscored by research which suggests that psychological abuse can be subtle in nature and characterized not only by the presence of certain behaviors but the *absence* of others. Murphy's construct of Hostile Withdrawal, which consists of withholding of emotional availability or contact in either a cold or punitive fashion, is a good one and in the tradition of psychodynamic theory of passive-aggressive behavior. Reliable assessment of this type of construct, however, requires careful attention to historical and contextual information in the relationship as well as the concurrent assessment of potentially difficult to access issues of motivation or intent. For example, a victim who has become emotionally withdrawn from a relationship due to a history of abusive treatment may be engaging in post-traumatic or self-protective behavior as opposed to a form of hostile withdrawal or emotional abandonment.

When issues of intent and motivation are invoked as constructs important to the understanding of psychological abuse, we begin to look inside "the black box" of personal attitude and emotion.

While some applied researchers have advocated the incorporation of anger and hostility in a comprehensive model of etiology and intervention for domestically violent individuals (Dutton, Saunders, Starzomski & Bartholomew, 1994; Maiuro, Cahn, & Vitaliano, 1986; Maiuro, Cahn, Vitaliano, Wagner, & Zegree, 1988; Maiuro, Hager, Lin, & Olsen, in press; Maiuro, Vitaliano, & Cahn, 1987) other writers have questioned the relevance of such emotions and attitudes to battering (Gondolf, 1986). They argue that anger is an emotion rather than a behavior and may not be related to the behavior of battering in some domestically violent men. However, one would expect that as the field turns its attention to psychological and emotional abuse, the role of anger may be more completely understood as an important component of some forms of psychological abuse, a potentially abusive means of achieving dominance, power, and control, and an important precursor to some forms of physical violence.

Although the potential escalating quality of domestic violence has been repeatedly documented in the literature, few studies have detailed the factors associated with this progression. The inclusion of measures of psychological aggression as well as the attitudes, and emotional and social environmental context that propel this process may give us insight into how this happens. For example, it would be interesting to see what forms of psychological abuse constitute the tension-building phase of the cycle of violence. Similarly studies of psychological abuse may help us understand the tendency for physical abuse to escalate in some cases of domestic violence while in others it does not. Such studies are needed if the field is to ever realize the goal of primary or secondary prevention as opposed to the current focus upon tertiary levels of prevention and intervention that is all too late in the game for many victimized partners.

All too often victim and perpetrator databases are collected in isolation. While case management and safety precautions may indeed require the separation of domestic partners in applied research settings, the relative dearth of couple data sets significantly limits our scientific understanding of the dynamics of psychological abuse in domestic violence. This is not surprising given the fact that domestic violence, after all, is a form of *interpersonal* violence. Relatively absent from the present compilation is a study of perceived psychological abuse from the perspective of the perpetrator.

While we should be mindful that serious and injurious forms of physical violence are more frequently perpetrated by men, and that a significant amount of violence by women is in self-defense or retaliatory in nature, less is known about the relative degree to which psychological and emotional tactics are employed by men and women in domestically violent relationships. In a recent study, Harned (in press) assessed a large sample of dating partners, taking care to assess not only the type of abuse perpetrated and received, but the motives and outcomes reported by participants. While women were more likely to be the recipients of sexual victimization and suffered more severe impact from physical violence, rates of violence reportedly engaged in for purposes of self-defense and psychological abuse were similar across genders. Although the generalizability of these findings to severe, clinical, and adjudicated cases of domestic violence remains an open question, the data are of pertinent interest given the large sample and methodology employed.

As in the case of studies of physical violence, careful attention must be given to interpreting data on men and women within a violence, power, and gender sensitive context to avoid blaming female victims for "psychologically" provoking their own victimization. On the other hand, the conduct and discussion of such research will probably never exist without some level of healthy controversy. As long as care is taken to collect couple data with the use of protocols which ensure the safety of victims, and the use of sophisticated designs and interpretative frames of reference, it should help advance our understanding and intervention for both men and women afflicted with the problem of domestic violence and abuse.

ROLAND D. MAIURO

REFERENCES

Blumenthal, D. R., Neeman, J., & Murphy, C. M. (1998). Lifetime exposure to interparental physical and verbal aggression and symptom expression in college students. *Violence and Victims, 13,* 175-196.

Burman, B., Margolin, G., & John, R. S. (1993). America's angriest home videos: Behavioral contingencies observed in home reenactments of marital conflict. Special Section: Couples and couple therapy. *Journal of Consulting & Clinical Psychology, 61,* 28-39.

Coker, A. L., Smith, P. H., Bethee, L., King, M. R., & McKeown, R. E. (2000). Physical health consequences of physical and psychological intimate partner abuse. *Archives of Family Medicine, 9,* 451-457.

Coleman, D. H., & Straus, M. A. (1986). Marital power, conflict, and violence in a nationally representative sample of American couples. *Violence and Victims, 1,* 141-157.

Dutton, D. G., & Painter, S. (1993). Emotional attachments in abusive relationships: A test of traumatic bonding theory. *Violence and Victims, 8,* 105-120.

Dutton, D. G., Saunders, K., Starzomski, A., & Bartholomew, K. (1994). Intimacy anger and insecure attachment as precursors of abuse in intimate relationships. *Journal of Applied Social Psychology, 24,* 1367-1386.

Follingstad, D. R., Rutledge, L. L., Berg, B. J., Hause, E. S., & Polek, D. S. (1990). The role of emotional abuse in physically abusive relationships. *Journal of Family Violence, 5,* 107-120.

Gondolf, E., & Russell, D. (1986). The case against anger control treatment for batterers. *Response, 9,* 2-5.

Graham, D. L. R., with Rawlings, E. I., & Rigsby, R. (1994). *Loving to survive: Sexual terror, men's violence and women's lives.* New York: University Press.

Hamby, S. L., Poindexter, V. C., & Gray-Little, B. (1996). Four measures of partner violence: Construct similarity and classification differences. *Journal of Marriage and the Family, 58,* 127-139.

Harned, M. (in press). Abused women or abused men? An examination of the context and outcomes of dating violence. *Violence and Victims.*

Hudson, W. W., & McIntosh, S. R. (1981). The assessment of spouse abuse: Two quantifiable dimensions. *Journal of Marriage and the Family, 43,* 873-885.

Koss, M. P., Goodman, L. A., Browne, A., Fitzgerald, L. F., Keita, G. P., & Russo, N. P. (1994). *No safe haven: Male violence against women at home, at work, and in the community.* Washington, DC: American Psychological Association.

Leonard, K. E., & Senchak, M. (1996). Prospective prediction of husband marital aggression within newlywed couples. *Journal of Abnormal Psychology, 105,* 368-380.

Maiuro, R. D., Cahn, T. S., & Vitaliano, P. P. (1986). Assertiveness and hostility in domestically violent men. *Violence and Victims, 1,* 279-289.

Maiuro, R. D., Cahn, T. S., Vitaliano, P. P., Wagner, B. C., & Zegree, J. B. (1988). Anger, hostility, and depression in domestically violent versus generally assaultive men and nonviolent control subjects. *Journal of Consulting and Clinical Psychology, 56,* 17-23.

Maiuro, R. D., Hager, T., Lin, H., & Olsen, N. (in press). Are current state standards for domestically violent perpetrator treatment adequately informed by research: A question of questions? *Journal of Abuse, Maltreatment, and Trauma.*

Maiuro, R. D., Vitaliano, P. P., & Cahn, T. S. (1987). Assertiveness deficits and hostility in domestically violent men. *Violence and Victims, 2,* 166-178.

Marshall, L. L. (1994). Physical and psychological abuse. In W. R. Cupach & B. H. Spitzberg (Eds.), *The dark side of interpersonal communication* (pp. 281-311). Hillsdale, NJ: Lawrence Erlbaum Associates.

Marshall, L. L. (1996). Psychological abuse of women: Six distinct clusters. *Journal of Family Violence, 11,* 369-399.

Murphy, C. M., & O'Leary, K. D. (1989). Psychological aggression predicts physical aggression in early marriage. *Journal of Consulting and Clinical Psychology, 57,* 579-582.

O'Leary, K. D., Malone, J., & Tyree, A. (1994). Physical aggression in early marriage: Prerelationship and relationship effects. *Journal of Consulting and Clinical Psychology, 62,* 594-602.

Rosenbaum, A., & Maiuro, R. D. (1989). Eclectic approaches in working with men who batter (pp. 165-195). In P. L. Caesar & L. K. Hamberger (Eds.). *Treating men who batter: Theory, practice, and programs.* New York: Springer Publishing.

Tolman, R. M. (1989). The development of a measure of psychological maltreatment of women by their male partners. *Violence and Victims, 4,* 159-177.

Walker, L. E. A. (1994). *Abused women and survivor therapy: A practical guide for the psychotherapist.* Washington, DC: APA Press.

Williams, O. J., & Becker, R. L. (1994). Domestic partner abuse treatment programs and cultural competence: The results of a national survey. *Violence and Victims, 9,* 287-296.

Acknowledgments

The work presented in Chapter 1 was supported in part by NIMH grants MH57985 and MH47801.

Portions of Chapter 2 were presented at the 5th International Family Violence Research Conference in Durham, New Hampshire in June, 1997.

Chapter 4 was originally presented at the 4th International Family Violence Research Conference, Durham, NH, July, 1995. Support for the study was provided by the Family Research Laboratory of the University of New Hampshire and NIMH grant 5-T32-MH15161.

Research presented in Chapter 5 was partially funded by the University of Cincinnati Center for Women's Studies.

Research presented in Chapter 6 was supported by grants from the National Center for Nursing Research and the Centers for Disease Control.

Research presented in Chapter 8 was supported in part by National Institute on Alcohol Abuse and Alcoholism (NIAAA) Grant AA09224-02S1.

The study outlined in Chapter 9 was funded by grant #R49/CCR610508 from the National Center for Injury Prevention and Control of the Centers for Disease Control and Prevention. Initial examination of subtle and overt psychological abuse was funded by grant #R29MH44217 from the National Institute of Mental Health.

Part I

Measurement Issues

Chapter 1

Psychological Abuse: A Variable Deserving Critical Attention in Domestic Violence

K. Daniel O'Leary

I n the domestic violence field there has been general agreement that research and public policy should focus on reduction of physical aggression. That focus has been reasonable since fear of physical abuse and the injury resulting therefrom has been presumed to be greater than the effects of psychological abuse. Since 1979, when the seminal books of Walker (1979) and Straus, Gelles, and Steinmetz (1979) appeared, the focus in domestic violence has been on physical aggression. Yet in 1979 Walker wrote as follows in *The Battered Woman:* "Most of the women in this project describe incidents involving psychological humiliation and verbal harassment as their worst battering experiences, whether or not they have been physically abused" (p. xv). The sample used by Walker was "a self-referred volunteer one." As depicted in the introduction to the book, the sample came from the New Brunswick, New Jersey, area, from Denver, and from England, where Walker visited "refuges for battered women." Walker went on to state that "the women were not randomly selected, and they cannot be considered a legitimate data base from which to make specific generalizations." Consequently, Walker attempted not to use any statistics throughout the book to analyze any of the data. Nonetheless, her book was one of the first descriptive analyses of domestic violence, and Walker portrayed the psychological aggression in a manner that was as important as the physical aggression.

In a now classic book on domestic violence, *Behind Closed Doors* (1979), Straus, Gelles, and Steinmetz reported on their interviews with 2,143 individuals and their domestic violence experiences. As Straus and colleagues stated, when they began their work in the late 1970s, there was no book on physical violence between spouses. The book was written to be understood by the general public and therefore technical presentation and methodological details were avoided. With that caveat, the thrust of the text was on physical violence.

> Drive down any street in America. More than one household in six has been the scene of a spouse striking his or her partner last year. Three American households in five (which have children living at home), have reverberated with the sounds of parents hitting their children. Where there is more than one child in the home, three in five are the scenes of violence between siblings. Overall, every other house in America is the scene of family violence at least once a year. (p. 3)

Physical abuse was documented in this book in a fashion that it had never been portrayed before. Straus and his colleagues had a randomly selected sample of individuals who were in intact families. Interviews were completed with 65% of the individuals identified. Moreover, a measure of a number of specifically physically aggressive behaviors that might be engaged in by husbands and wives was utilized to determine the prevalence of physical aggression. Approximately 12 % of men and 12 % of women reported that they had engaged in physically aggressive behaviors against their partners in the past year. Verbal aggression also was addressed in the book (pp. 167–169, 173), but it was addressed largely in the context of the then popular theory of catharsis. (At that time, foam rubber baseball bats were advertised in the American Psychological Association's *Monitor* and in *Human Behavior* for getting rid of aggressive impulses.)

The book by Straus and his colleagues has certainly been one of the most influential in the field of family violence. By providing a measure of physical aggression in intimate relations, it gave others a means of conducting research on heretofore ignored subjects. The Conflict Tactics Scales also contained a measure of psychological aggression, but it received less emphasis—as it probably should have at the time, given the neglect of partner assault as a bonafide form of assault by the criminal justice system. At this point, however, it is time to recognize the importance of psychological aggression in its own right, and fortunately, several recent chapters have begun to address psychological abuse in marriage (e.g., Murphy & Cascardi, 1993; O'Leary & Jouriles, 1994). In this chapter, data will be presented to provide documentation for the reliability and validity of the construct of psychological aggression. In doing so, I will provide evidence for the following positions:

1. Psychological aggression can be measured reliably.
2. When physical aggression occurs, it often is preceded by psychological aggression.

3. Psychological aggression often has effects that are as deleterious as those of physical aggression.
4. Psychological aggression can be defined in a manner that allows for reliable assessment and use of this construct in both mental health and legal settings.

PSYCHOLOGICAL AGGRESSION CAN BE MEASURED RELIABLY

There are a number of measures of psychological aggression that have reasonable internal consistency and that have important correlates with other variables of interest to researchers and clinicians addressing problems of partner abuse. Those measures of psychological aggression will be reviewed herein in the order in which they were published.

Conflict Tactics Scale. In 1979, Straus developed the Conflict Tactics Scale designed to evaluate the different tactics that might be used by partners in resolving a conflict. As noted earlier, the major thrust of the research using the CTS has been about physical violence, and, indeed, the most recent major text about that work was titled *Physical Violence in American Families* (Straus & Gelles, 1992). Included in the CTS, however, was a six-item psychological aggression scale. The internal consistency of the psychological aggression scale was .80 for husband to wife aggression and .79 for wife to husband aggression (Straus, 1990). Items on the psychological aggression scale include both verbal and nonverbal acts. Items of that scale are the following: (1) insulted or swore at her/him; (2) sulked or refused to talk about an issue; (3) stomped out of the room or house or yard; (4) did or said something to spite her/him; (5) threatened to hit or throw something at him or her; and (6) threw, smashed, hit or kicked something. As Straus (1990) noted, the items on this scale include verbal and nonverbal acts which symbolically hurt the other or the use of threats to hurt the other. Thus, the scale certainly is a measure of psychological aggression, and the revised CTS uses the label psychological aggression for this construct (Straus, Hamby, Boney-McCoy, & Sugarman, 1995).

Although the primary focus was initially on physical violence in families, Straus and his colleagues also showed that the more psychologically aggressive partners are to one another, the more likely they are to be physically aggressive (Straus, 1974; Straus & Smith, 1990). Moreover, the more psychologically aggressive parents are toward their children, the more likely they were to be physically abusive to the children. Such findings argued against the then popular catharsis model of coping with family problems (Berkowitz, 1973). Moreover, Suitor, Pillemer, and Straus (1990) reported that verbal aggression declines monotonically across the life course.

Index of Spouse Abuse. Hudson and McIntosh (1981) published one of the first measures of partner abuse called the Index of Spouse Abuse (ISA), which was intended to assess both psychological and physical abuse of women. The measure was developed using both undergraduate and graduate female college students at the University of Hawaii as well as a comparison group of abused and nonabused women. The ISA is a 30-item scale in which the respondent rates the extent to which a partner engages in the various behaviors (from 1 [never] to 5 [very frequently]). A severity of physical abuse index and a severity of psychological abuse index are obtained. The psychological and physical abuse scales of the ISA had internal consistencies greater than .90 (Campbell, Campbell, King, Parker, & Ryan, 1994; Hudson & McIntosh, 1981) and, as would be expected, the correlations of psychological and physical abuse were high (r = .66; Campbell et al., 1994; Hudson & McIntosh, 1981, r = .86). Factor analyses by Campbell and associates suggest different loadings of the ISA items of the physical aggression factor than the original Hudson and McIntosh (1981) analyses. The factor analyses also revealed a psychological abuse factor and a new factor that essentially comprised a second psychological abuse scale that Campbell and colleagues felt was a measure of domination and control.

In 1990, Hudson further developed the ISA with two separate scales, a psychological and a physical abuse scale. Each scale comprises 25 items with scores that range from 0–100. In 1994, Alta, Hudson, and McSweeney partly validated the scales and determined cutoff scores for determination of probable abuse. In brief, the ISA is a measure of psychological abuse that is internally consistent and factorially sound. Research by Campbell and colleagues (1994) indicates that measures developed with one racial group (unspecified Hawaiian sample) may not have the same psychometric properties in another population (African American). Nonetheless, the ISA has been given some validation support from clinical interviews by McFarlane, Parker, Soeken, and Bullock (1992). More specifically, physical abuse and psychological abuse were assessed with the ISA in a population of women identified as abused in a brief 5-item questionnaire used in an interview format. Moreover, the ISA physical abuse scale was found to correlate .77 with a dangerousness measure, and the psychological abuse scale was found to correlate .66 with a dangerousness measure (Campbell et al., 1994).

Spouse Specific Aggression and Assertion. In 1986, O'Leary and Curley published the Spouse Specific Aggression Scale (SSAgg) and the Spouse Specific Assertion Scale (SSAss). In line with the Zeitgeist of the times, the scales were developed to differentially assess psychological aggression and assertion. In the mid-1970s, assertion books were so popular that the there was a guide to the selection of assertion books (Landau, 1976), and assertion training had been recommended for abused women though we had expressed concern that assertion training, if not very carefully implemented, could place abused women at risk (O'Leary, Curley, Rosenbaum, & Clark, 1985). There are 12 items that assess psychological aggression, and 9 of those items were adapted from the Buss-Durkee Hostility Inventory to reflect spouse-specific aggression (Buss & Durkee, 1957). In addition, 17 items were developed to assess assertion toward a partner (either male or female). The initial pool of items was rated by a panel of eight graduate-student judges who classified the items as describing an assertive response, an aggressive response, or neither. Interrater reliability of .86 was obtained on the final version of the scale. Internal consistency as measured by alpha was .82 for the spouse specific psychological aggression scale and .87 for the spouse specific assertion scale. In comparisons of groups of men and women hypothesized to have different levels of psychological aggression, physically abusive men reported more psychological aggression toward their partners than happily married men and than discordant nonphysically abusive men. In addition, the abusive men had lower spouse specific assertion scores than the happily married men but not than discordant nonabusive men. Women in physically abusive relationships reported more spouse-specific psychological aggression toward their spouses than the satisfactorily married women, but the discordant women did not report more spouse-specific aggression than the satisfactorily married women (O'Leary & Curley, 1986). More recently, spouse specific psychological aggression has been shown to characterize physically abusive men who were mandated to treatment as well as male volunteers who were not physically abusive (Rathus, O'Leary, & Meyer, 1997). Further, spouse specific aggression was one of the best differentiators of physically aggressive, discordant men from nonphysically aggressive discordant men (Boyle & Vivian, 1996).

Psychological Maltreatment of Women Inventory. In 1989, Tolman developed a scale called Psychological Maltreatment of Women Inventory (PMWI), an instrument to assess the manner in which a male partner controls a female partner. Participants are asked to indicate how often certain behaviors occurred within the last 2 years. The scale was developed with 407 batterers and 207 women at intake for a domestic violence program (though the men and women were generally not related). As a consequence of the context of the subject acquisition, the PMWI contains items that reflect quite controlling behaviors. For example, the dominance-isolation scale includes the following items: limited her access to telephone; prevented or limited her use of the car; limited her access to money; asked her to account for her time and report where she had been. The emotional verbal scale includes items such as the following: yelled and screamed; called her names; told partner that her feelings were crazy; insulted or shamed her in front of others. The PMWI was developed to be compatible with the Conflict Tactics Scale by Straus (1979) and the Index of Spouse Abuse (ISA) by Hudson and McIntosh (1981). Tolman wanted to have a measure that could be used to obtain men's reports of their own psychological aggression and he wanted to sample a broader range of psychologically abusive behaviors, especially of the monitoring and isolation qualities. Indeed some of the items in the PMWI were modified from the nonphysical abuse scale of the ISA of Hudson and McIntosh. Tolman excluded items that would assess behaviors described as psychological maltreatment, if those items had a direct physical component (such as interrupting sleep, forcing sex) or items that included threats of harm, since such items are covered in measures such as the CTS.

Factor analyses of an original pool of 58 items yielded a Psychological Maltreatment of Women Inventory with two factors whether using reports by men or women: an emotional-verbal abuse factor and a dominance-isolation factor. The first factor contains 28 items; the second has 20 items. As might be expected, the factors were highly correlated for both men ($r = .73$) and women ($r = .74$). While the men's and women's reports are not directly comparable as the men and women were from different relationships, in the populations used by Tolman the women's reports of the extent of maltreatment were considerably higher on both the dominance-isolation and the emotional-verbal subscales. Internal consistency of the dominance-isolation scale was reported for male respondents to be .91; it was .93 for the emotional-verbal abuse scale. For women reporting about their husbands dominance/isolation, the alpha was .94; for women reporting about their emotional-verbal abuse, the alpha was .92.

Another study compared violent men, using the two scales of the PMWI, to men in discordant nonviolent relationships, and happily married men. The two clinical groups had higher scores on the emotional/verbal abuse scale than the happily married men, but, contrary to predictions, they did not differ from one another (Rathus, O'Leary, & Meyer, 1997). Similarly, the two clinical groups had higher scores on the dominance/isolation scale than the happily married group, but they did not differ from one another. Physically abusive men in this study had to have at least two mild acts or one severe act of husband-to-wife physical aggression within the past year. They had an average of 7.5 acts in the year ($SD = 5.3$). The modal number of physically aggressive acts was three. With this sample of men who were physically aggressive toward their partners but had been volunteers for treatment or mandated to treatment, the levels of dominance and isolation differed from those of Tolman's sample of men in a group for batterers. The mean score of the men in the Tolman sample on dominance-isolation subscale was 43.3 ($SD = 15.8$) out of a possible range of 20 to 100. In contrast, the mean of the distressed, violent group on this scale was 29.6 ($SD = 5.5$). The sample differences on this variable are clearly a matter of importance, and, in accord with suggestions by a number of researchers in this area, it may be necessary to delineate types of men (and women) in different kinds of aggressive relationships (Hamberger & Hastings, 1986; Holtzworth-Munroe & Stuart, 1994; O'Leary, 1993).

A brief version of the PMWI contains two 7-item scales of dominance-isolation and verbal-emotional abuse (Tolman, 1999). Both of these scales successfully discriminated between three groups: (1) battered, maritally distressed, (2) maritally distressed but not physically abused, (3) maritally satisfied and not physically abused. Women were recruited for this study from an agency for battered women and from newspaper announcements. The dominance-isolation scale had an internal consistency of .88 and the verbal-emotional abuse scale had an internal consistency of .92. Factor loadings of the abbreviated scale showed that the factor structure was consistent with the factor structure of the larger scale (PMWI).

Moreover, the battered women scored significantly higher on the two abbreviated scales than the women in the other two groups: the maritally distressed but not physically abused women and the maritally satisfied women.

Additional analyses of the battered women who sought services from an agency for battered women and those who were not treatment seeking revealed that it was the women seeking help from an agency for battered women who differed on the maltreatment scales from the women in the relationships that were distressed but nonviolent. However, women in physically abusive relationships that were not treatment-seeking differed only on one of four measures, the short dominance scale, from the women in distressed nonviolent relationships. These findings seem to echo the need to distinguish between people in different types of physically abusive relationships, a point made by Hamberger and Hastings (1986), Holtzworth-Munroe and Stuart (1994), and O'Leary, (1993).

Index of Psychological Abuse. In 1991, Sullivan, Parisian, and Davidson presented a poster at the American Psychological Association in which they presented material on the development of a measure of psychological abuse. The 33-item scale was designed to measure the amount of ridicule, harassment, isolation, and control a woman experienced. Women indicated on a 4-point scale how frequently they experienced a particular form of abuse. The scale was intended to be used in both dating and marital relationships, and it was piloted in two research projects, one involving dating aggression in college students and one involving the follow-up of women who had utilized a battered women's shelter. Items were subjected to a principal components factor analysis which yielded six subscales with varied numbers of items listed in brackets: (1) Criticism and Ridicule [9], (2) Social Isolation and Control [5], (3) Threats and Violence [4], (4) Emotional Withdrawal [3], (5) Manipulation [3], and (6) Emotional Callousness [3]. The six scales were then developed with the dating population and later used with women from domestic violence shelters. Alphas for the six scales ranged from .68 to .93, and correlations among the measures ranged from .52 to .83, with 9 of the 15 correlations being higher than .70. While the correlations suggest strong overlap among the types of psychological abuse, there was some evidence that certain types of psychological abuse had greater associations with some dependent measures than others. For example, Criticism and Ridicule had the strongest associations with physical abuse, namely .61. All six scales had relatively low but significant correlations with depressive symptomatology, namely, all about .30 to .35. In brief, the Index of Psychological Abuse is a scale that could be used as is or developed further, depending upon the type of psychological abuse one wishes to assess.

The Abusive Behavior Inventory (ABI). In 1992, Shepard and Campbell used feminist theory to assess a wide range of abusive behaviors. Psychological abuse was seen as a means of establishing power and control over the victim. One hundred men and 78 women were divided equally into groups of abusers/abused and nonabusers/nonabused (the method of differentiating the criterion groups was not specified). All men were part of a chemical dependency program located in a Veteran's Administration hospital; the women were married to these men. The ABI is a 30-item inventory using a 5-point Likert scale (1 = no psychological abuse to 5 = very frequent psychological abuse) to measure the frequency of 20 psychologically abusive behaviors and 10 physically abusive behaviors during a 30-month period. The scale was developed for the purpose of evaluating a domestic abuse program.

Alpha coefficients for the four groups ranged from .70 to .92. As predicted, the men in the abuse group had higher scores on the psychological and physical abuse items than the nonabusive men. Physical abuse items had more consistent correlations with the total physical subscale than psychological abuse items had with their total psychological abuse subscale score. More specifically, 7 of the 20 psychological abuse items for men had higher correlations with the physical abuse subscale than with the psychological abuse subscale (e.g., items reflecting economic abuse, isolation, threats of force, and reckless driving). As the authors note, these results point to the need for replication and extension of measurement models with diverse populations. This is especially important because the way in which one should score psychological and physical aggression factors is often unclear when the items load on a factor other than the one hypothesized.

This study by Shepard and Campbell had one feature which is especially laudatory, namely, the use of the clinician's assessment of psychological abuse and the client's assessment of abuse. While details of the specific means of obtaining such ratings were not described, the need for clinical validation such as this is important. The correlations of the clinicians ratings with the Psychological Abuse Subscale were .20 for men's reports of the behavior and .25 for women's reports of the behavior. Unfortunately, the correlations were not reported for the four groups, and even the reported correlations are very modest. However, this is the only attempt to provide clinician's ratings of abuse in any of the psychological abuse measurement studies reported herein. Finally, it was a surprise to me that the mean ratings of psychological abuse were so low for the abuse group, namely 2.1 as reported by men and 2.8 as reported by women on a 5-point Likert scale for 20 psychological abuse items (range of scores could be from 1 to 5). Such data suggest that even when using the women's reports, men are seen as rarely engaging in the behaviors described. However, even the women's reports of the men's physical abuse were only 1.8. Since it is unclear how often these psychologically abusive behaviors are engaged in by men in various samples, especially highly controlling behaviors, it will be helpful for all investigators to describe the frequencies of all of the specific items in the scale.

Severity of Violence Against Women. In 1992(a), Marshall published her Severity of Violence Against Women Scales. The scales were developed with college females (N = 707) who rated 46 various acts of aggression in terms of seriousness, abusiveness, violence, and threatening nature. The acts were to be rated "if a man carried out these acts with a woman." Community women ($N = 208$) also rated the acts in terms of seriousness, aggressiveness, and abusiveness. When the students rated the violence, nine factors emerged ranging from symbolic violence and threats of mild violence to serious violence, and sexual violence. Because of problems of very low response rates of community women (16%), community women were not asked to evaluate the acts of aggression using the same descriptors as the students, and thus the factor analyses based on the community sample are not comparable to those of the students. However, a second order factor analysis revealed two factors that basically represented a psychological aggression factor and a physical/sexual violence factor. The acts represented in the Marshall scales represent detailed behaviors of different levels of psychological and physical aggression, and the use of the items and/or scales with populations of abused and maritally discordant populations would be valuable. Basically, the scales represent a beginning point for researchers interested in mapping the typologies of psychological abuse. Marshall extended her research on the assessment of psychological abuse of women by men to include a measure of psychological abuse by women of men (Marshall, 1992b). The types of violence measured were threats of mild violence, threats of moderate violence, and threats of severe violence. As was the case with the development of the violence against women scales, a college student sample and community sample of males rated acts of violence as if a woman engaged in the acts of violence against a man. That is, the acts represent behaviors that might be engaged in by women. Thus, replication and extension of this work with clinical populations is certainly in order.

The Measurement of Wife Abuse (MWA). Rodenburg and Fantuzzo (1993) published The Measurement of Wife Abuse, a measure "developed to improve upon previously constructed instruments, mainly by using empirical methods of construction." The subjects in the study were abused women, most of whom came from an outpatient clinic or a battered women's shelter. There were also some women who responded to radio and newspaper announcements about the study. To be included, a woman had to be physically abused at least three times, as assessed by the Conflict Tactics Scale. The measure was a revision of an unpublished master's thesis (Lambert & Fantuzzo, 1988). The MWA examines frequency of different kinds of abuse based on number of acts within a 6-month period as well as the emotional consequences experienced by the victim. Items for the scale were taken from Rhodes (1985) who compiled the items from over 250 restraining orders or legal documents which contained descriptions of abuse by partners. Card-sorting procedures were used initially to sort items into categories: (1) psychological abuse, (2) physical abuse, (3) sexual abuse, and (4) verbal abuse. Because the focus in this chapter is on psychological abuse, that 15-item measure will be discussed here. Severity ratings based on a 4-point scale were subject to a confirmatory factor analysis. Concurrent validity was assessed by measures of association with the CTS. The psychological abuse measure contained 15 items that involved restriction (disabled car, locked in, electricity off) whereas the verbal abuse items were about verbal denigration (told ugly, told stupid, called bitch). Contrary to the author's expectations, the four factors of the MWA were all significantly intercorrelated, at approximately equal rates (all between .41 and .56). The psychological abuse measure and the verbal abuse measure correlated .46. Seventy-five percent of the items met a correlation criterion of .30 with its hypothesized factor. One item, attempted suicide, had a loading of less than .20. Thus, the psychological abuse scale has 14 items that have reasonable loadings. The correlations of the psychological abuse scale of the MWA with the Psychological Abuse and the Physical Aggression Scale of the CTS were .23 and .22, respectively. These correlations, while significant ($N = 132$), indicate relatively little overlap in the variance accounted for in the measures. Thus, while there is some evidence of convergence of measures, the validity of the psychological abuse scale of the MWA needs to be better established, or it would be important to provide evidence about why the MWA should not be associated with measures of abuse developed by others.

The Dominance Scale. In 1996, Hamby published The Dominance Scale, which appears to measure three different forms of dominance: Authority, Restrictiveness, and Disparagement. Each of these forms of dominance were seen as one kind of deviation from an egalitarian relationship. Hamby conceptualized the above three forms of dominance as "causes of violence, including physical and psychological aggression, not as violence in and of itself." The scale was developed with a college student population of whom only 14% were married, and thus the population was essentially about dating relationships. There were 51 males and 80 females attending one of two colleges in the Northeast. Participants were recruited through sociology and justice studies courses. Because of the small sample, factor analyses were not conducted on the full Dominance item pool. Instead, separate factor analyses were conducted for each theoretical scale to assess communalities. A one factor solution was obtained in each case. Restrictiveness and disparagement were uncorrelated ($r = .03$); authority and restrictiveness had a correlation of .38; authority and disparagement had a correlation of .58. According to Hamby, the pattern of correlations was not significantly different for males and females. Restrictiveness was significantly correlated with physical aggression and injury, but authority and disparagement were not. All three components of the Dominance Scale were significantly correlated with reports of one's own psychological aggression. As noted by Hamby, the results of studies using authority or decision-making measures as a means of assessing dominance, may not be very closely related to partner violence. Based on her work, restrictive control may be more closely related to partner violence than authoritarian control. While the Hamby Dominance Scale is based on a relatively small college sample, the work raises important questions about dominance and the need to separate components of this construct.

Hamby argued that the Dominance Scale was not a measure of psychological aggression but instead a predictor of such aggression. However, the three dominance constructs all correlated, albeit moderately, with self-reported and partner-reported psychological aggression as measured by the revised Conflict Tactics Scale. Thus, the Dominance Scale can be interpreted as one form of psychological aggression, or at least a construct whose components are all significantly related to psychological aggression.

In summary, there are eight measures of psychological aggression that have both internal consistency and demonstrable construct validity. The following investigators all have measures of psychological abuse: Hamby (1996); Hudson and McIntosh (1981); Marshall (1992); O'Leary and Curley, (1986); Rodenberg and Fantuzzo (1993); Shepard and Campbell (1992); Straus (1979); Tolman (1989). Each of the measures was designed for a somewhat different purpose, and thus each assesses psychological abuse somewhat differently. As data are presented on the three other major issues in this chapter, i.e., the temporal precedence of psychological to physical aggression, the impact of psychological and physical aggression, and a definition of partner abuse that could be used for clinical and legal purposes, additional research findings will be presented that further support the construct validity of various measures of psychological aggression since the aforementioned measures of psychological aggression have been used in a number of studies to be discussed later.

When Physical Aggression Occurs, It Is Often Preceded by Psychological/Verbal Aggression

In a longitudinal study of the etiology of partner violence, Murphy and O'Leary (1989) found that psychological aggression was a precursor of physical aggression in young couples. The young couples were engaged to be married within one month of the initial assessment. Couples were recruited from the community and were similar to the counties from which they were drawn in terms of age at first marriage and religious affiliation. The couples were almost exclusively White and had 14.5 years of education, 1.5 years more than the average for the local area. Two hundred and seventy-two couples participated at each assessment. Psychological aggression was measured by a combined score based on the CTS and the Spouse Specific Aggression Scale. These scores were transformed into Z scores and summed to form a composite index of psychological aggression. (The correlations between the two measures of psychological aggression at the initial assessment were .47 for men and .68 for women for the nonphysically aggressive subjects in this study.) Couples were selected for not having been physically aggressive to their partner in the past year or at any other time prior to the assessment of psychological aggression. The psychological aggression scores were used to predict the onset of the first acts of physical aggression (as reported by either the husband or the wife).

Across a 6-month period (from premarriage to 6 months after marriage), the lag correlations of psychological aggression and physical aggression (assessed dichotomously) were all significant. In predicting the husband's first instance of physical aggression, based on his self report, the correlation was .31; based on the wife's reports, the correlation was .19. In predicting wives' first instance of physical aggression, based on self-report, the correlation was .15. Based on partner report, the correlation was .32. With a lag of 12 months from 6 to 18 months into marriage, the correlations again were all significant and ranged from .29 to .34. The 18- to 30-month correlations were only significant for self-reports of psychological aggression and physical aggression.

As might be expected, cross-sectional associations were higher than the lag correlations. In predicting husbands' physical aggression, the correlations were .40, based on self-report and .33 based on partner report. In predicting wives' physical aggression, the correlations were .38 based on self-report and .40 based on partner report. Moreover, at 1 year, the correlations were again all significant and ranged from .33 to .41. At 30 months into marriage, three of the four correlations were significant.

In contrast to the consistent association across 6- and 12-month periods of psychological and physical aggression, general marital satisfaction was not predictive of later physical aggression. Only one of 23 longitudinal correlations was predictive of later physical aggression. The above results support the general model that psychologically coercive behaviors precede and predict the development of physically aggressive behavior in marriage (O'Leary, 1988). The importance of the negative interchanges and psychological aggression in the development of partner violence has been described clinically (e.g., Deschner, 1984), and this research supports the hypothesized progression from psychological to physical aggression in early marriage.

In a different analysis of the couples in the longitudinal research noted above, O'Leary, Malone, and Tyree (1994) showed that there were direct paths from psychological aggression to physical aggression. Psychological aggression, as assessed at 18 months by the Spouse Specific Aggression Scale (O'Leary & Curley, 1986), had a direct path to physical aggression for men at 30 months with a path coefficient of .36. For women, there was a similar direct path from psychological aggression at 18 months to physical aggression at 30 months with a path coefficient of .29. The results discussed here are based on predictions of physical aggression at 30 months, although this aggression may not have been the first reported act of physical aggression in the relationship. In addition, we were able to show that men and women who have aggressive and defensive personality characteristics and who are experiencing a lack of satisfaction with their partners tend to engage in psychological aggression against their partners. In turn, as noted above, the psychological aggression was a precursor of physical aggression. In terms of gender differences, for women, there was a significant path from marital discord to physical aggression that did not exist for men. As we stated in the publication of these results, "We suspect that this finding may reflect the greater importance of relationship factors for women than men. Women may be more frustrated by marital discord, and impulsive women may be more likely to re-engage their partners after discordant interactions—even through aggressive physical contact." In addition to what was initially stated, women's marital discord usually is lower than men's and they may be more responsive to slights and negative interactions that are not reflected directly in psychological aggression.

The Effects of Psychological Aggression are Often as Deleterious as Those of Physical Aggression

One of the first studies to address the comparative role of psychological and physical aggression was that of Folingstad, Rutledge, Berg, Hause, and Polek (1990). Two hundred thirty-four women were interviewed to assess the relationship of emotional abuse to physical abuse. The women all had some history of physical abuse. Approximately one quarter of the women (26%) had no physical abuse in their relationships within the past 2 years while the remainder were experiencing long-term, ongoing abuse. Most of the women reported being out of the relationship; 33 still remained in the relationship. Recruitment occurred via announcements in newspapers, radio, and television as well as flyers in prisons, the department of social services, and in a local shelter.

Six types of emotional abuse were assessed for their frequency and impact:

(1) threats of abuse
(2) ridicule
(3) jealousy
(4) threats to change marriage status
(5) restriction
(6) damage to property

The abuse with the highest negative impact was ridicule, and it was one of the three most frequent types of abuse. Forty-six percent of the sample rated emotional ridicule as the worst type of abuse, 15% of the sample rated threats of abuse as the worst type of abuse, and 14% rated jealousy as the worst type of abuse.

To address the question of the relative impact of emotional and physical abuse, subjects rated whether emotional or physical abuse had a more negative impact on them. Seventy-two percent of the women rated emotional abuse as having a more negative impact on them than the physical abuse. Of interest, the women who reported emotional abuse as worse than physical abuse experienced the same degree of severity of typical physical abuse and the same frequency of abusive incidents during the first 6 months and subsequent months of abuse. Approximately half of the sample (54%) could predict the physical abuse they might receive from the emotional abuse they received.

Threats of abuse and restriction of the woman were predictors of later physical violence. Using a regression analysis, it was determined that threat of abuse was a very strong predictor that physical abuse would follow.

Marshall (1992a) also addressed the issue of impact of psychologically and physically aggressive behaviors. Of special import for the discussion here, 707 college women rated 46 various aggressive behaviors on how serious, aggressive, abusive, violent, and threatening it would be "if a man did the act to a woman" on a 10-point scale. The women rated symbolically (psychologically) aggressive and physically aggressive acts with a woman. Moreover, they rated how much emotional or psychological harm each of the acts would have on a woman. For 11 of 12 items like those that appear on the CTS and are called minor violence, the emotional impact ratings for students were all numerically higher than the physical impact ratings. The same pattern held for a sample of community women. Eleven of 12 items had higher emotional impact ratings than physical impact ratings. Marshall's data can be addressed in another way, namely, to evaluate the emotional impact of symbolic and psychological violence and compare that to the emotional impact of actual behavioral acts of violence. Unfortunately, items assessing symbolic or psychological aggression did not correspond directly to the actual behavioral acts of aggression. More specifically, threats of certain behavior did not correspond to engaging in those specific behaviors. However, it is clear from the students' ratings of emotional impact that threats of moderate violence and acts of moderate violence had almost the identical impact rating, 7.1 and 7.0, respectively. Moreover, threats of serious violence and acts of serious violence also had almost the same emotional impact rating, namely, 8.5 and 9.0, respectively. Threats of minor violence and acts of minor violence had different emotional impact ratings with the behavioral acts of aggression having higher impact ratings than the threats of minor violence, 7.0 versus 4.6. It appears clear from these data that the emotional impact of psychological violence can often be as negative as the emotional impact of physical violence, though for some behaviors the emotional impact of engaging in the acts can have greater impact than the threats of such acts. The research by Marshall has one important limitation, namely, that actual violence was not being evaluated by the college students or the community women. The ratings were done in a hypothetical sense. More specifically, women were asked how they would feel if a male partner did each of the acts. Replication and extension of this work with battered women would be useful to arrive at estimates of comparative effects of psychological and physical aggression.

Aguilar and Nightingale (1994) assessed the association of physical, sexual, and emotional abuse with self-esteem in 48 battered women. Using cluster analyses, four clusters of negative experiences were associated with battering experiences, namely, physical abuse, controlling/emotional abuse, sexual/emotional abuse, and miscellaneous abuse. The physical abuse category was comprised of items like those on the CTS (Straus, 1979): e.g., pushed, hit with fist, hit with an object, pinched, slapped, and choked. In addition, one nonphysical abuse item, called derogatory names, clustered with the physical abuse items. The controlling/ emotional abuse items included the following: told whom you can speak to; told whom you can see; told you cannot work; told what you can do. The sexual emotional cluster included the following: sexually abused, treated like a servant, told you are stupid, told you are crazy, treated as a sex object.

There was a fourth cluster that included only two items: bit and told how money is to be spent. As was evident from the cluster analyzes, the items that are derived from the cluster analysis procedure are not the same items that one would make from a logical analysis of items. For example, a physical abuse cluster has a nonphysical abuse item "called derogatory names." The particular items that fall into a cluster depend upon the specific items that were used in the cluster analysis, and the specific items determine whether one can obtain a cluster that reflects single or logically consistent groupings. Though the clusters found in this research do not fit into neat logically consistent packages, they did have empirical associations with self-esteem that are of significance. More specifically, women with high scores on the controlling/emotionally abuse cluster had lower self-esteem scores. In contrast, there was no association of physical abuse and sexual abuse with self-esteem. Unexpectedly, the fourth cluster, which included two items, being bit and being told how money was to be spent was associated with high self-esteem scores. This latter finding does not fit any particular theoretical or clinical description of battered women and it seems inconsistent with other findings. Without more explanation of the reasons for the results in this sample and until there is an attempt to replicate this finding, it seems fruitless to spend time attempting to explain the seemingly anomalous result. On the other hand, in keeping with the results of several other studies herein, the authors found greater association of psychological abuse with low self-esteem of women than with physical abuse.

In related research with 56 young, newly married couples, investigators addressed the association of psychological and physical aggression with later marital satisfaction and stability. Psychological and physical aggression were assessed with the Conflict Tactics Scale (Lawrence & Bradbury, 1995). Marital deterioration was defined as marital discord (Locke-Wallace Marital Adjustment Test of < 80) or marital dissolution. Survival analysis was the method used to assess the relationship of psychological aggression to the maintenance of marital satisfaction (or to marital dissolution). Basically, in this case, the survival analysis was a plotting of the risk for marital failure (discord or instability) of each subgroup (nonaggressive, psychologically aggressive, and physically aggressive), given the percent of couples in that subgroup who failed up to that point. Surprisingly, 32% of the couples experienced marital dissolution within the first 4 years of marriage, and 57% of wives and 55% of men reported discord over the 4 years.

Let us first address the association of aggression of the husband and his wife's report of marital deterioration. Although 57% of the wives of nonaggressive husbands experienced deterioration in their marriages, a similar percentage of wives (63%)of psychologically aggressive husbands reported deterioration. Finally, 75% of the wives of physically aggressive husbands experienced deterioration. There were no differences across the three groups. When aggression as reported by the wives was the independent variable and husbands' marital deterioration the dependent variable, the levels of deterioration were as follows: 13% for the nonaggressive group; 53% for the psychologically aggressive group; 88% for the physically aggressive group. These differences were significant, and they suggest that women's psychological and physical aggression can have a definite negative effect on the marital satisfaction/stability of the husband.

The absolute numbers, and, in turn, the cell sizes in this study are small, and the results reported for husbands' marital deterioration were more predictable than was the case for wives. The results for marital deterioration of wives, given aggression of their husbands, were not as we would expect, but the absence of differences could have been due in large part to the high rates of marital deterioration of the women in the nonaggressive group, namely, 57%. That is, even wives of nonaggressive husbands experienced marital deterioration for reasons that are not clear, and this high rate of deterioration made it difficult to detect differences across the groups.

Using a different design, Christian-Herman, O'Leary, and Avery-Leaf (in press) assessed the role of severe negative events in marriage on depression in women by interviewing the women within 1 month after a severe negative marital event. Women were recruited who had no history of a depressive episode in order to minimize the confound of past depression increasing the risk of later episodes. The sample of 50 women with no prior history of depression was recruited from a group of 273 women who responded to a newspaper advertisement. The types of events reported by the larger sample were comparable to those reported by the 50 subjects; the three most common negative marital events were as follows: (1) threat or actual separation/divorce, (2) affair or belief that an affair is ongoing, and (3) acts of physical aggression. Ratings of negative events were made by experienced marital researchers/therapists with a mean of 10 years of experience. Only 3% of the respondents reported a specific event which they perceived as severely negative but that was not judged to be negative by the outside raters. Those subjects were excluded. Thirty-eight percent of the women met diagnostic criteria for Major Depressive Episode when they were administered the SCID approximately 2 to 4 weeks after the occurrence of the severe negative marital event. This rate can be compared to the incidence rate of 2% reported by Eaton, Kramer, Anthony, Dryman, Shapiro, and Locke (1989) for women age 18-44 in the NIMH Epidemiological Catchment Area study. Thus, the negative marital event appeared to be a cause of the depression in a very significant percentage of these women. When a comparison was made about the most frequent types of negative marital events and the depression rates in those groups, the rates were as follows: (1) threats or actual separation/divorce: 63%; (2) perception that an affair was ongoing: 36%;

(3) physical aggression: 10%. Results from a Chi-square analysis indicated that there were higher rates of depression in the first two groups than in the physical aggression groups. These findings were a surprise to us, but led us to conclude that issues of loss were more likely to lead to depression than problems of physical aggression. Nonetheless, the rate of having a major depressive episode was approximately five times higher than the ECA incidence rates for depression, suggesting that physical aggression also increases the likelihood of having a major depressive episode in women who have never been depressed before. Overall, the results indicate that threats or actual separation/divorce or believing that an affair was ongoing placed women at higher risk for a major depressive episode than having been the victim of some act(s) of physical aggression by the partner.

A direct comparison of the effects of physical and psychological aggression was made by assessing impact ratings in a sample of couples in which both spouses reported physical aggression (Vivian & Langhinrichsen-Rohling, 1994). Aggression was defined as mutually agreed upon bidirectional aggression in a sample of 57 couples. This sample represented 39% of the total clinic sample of 145 couples who had sought marital therapy at the University Marital Therapy Clinic at Stony Brook. Physical aggression was reported to have occurred in 77% of the population of couples overall who came to the clinic. Impact ratings were made with a 1–7 range, with 1 being extremely negative and 7 being extremely positive. For wives, the impact of physical aggression was 1.94 while the impact of psychological aggression was 1.75. The second anchor point (2) on the scale was "quite negative," so that one can see that physical and psychological aggression both clearly have a negative impact. The impact of psychological abuse on women was greater than that for men, but upon further examination, it was seen that the difference was a function of one group of highly victimized women. Indeed, the mean ratings for impact of psychological aggression for men and women were identical except for a group of couples where the woman was highly victimized physically but the husband reported only mild to moderate physical victimization. The two groups in which the ratings were identical for men and women were in a group of couples in which both the men and women engaged in low levels of physical aggression and a smaller group in which the husband was highly physically victimized. When depressive symptomatology was assessed, the levels were found to be similar across groups and the depressive symptomatology scores were not different across men and women. The mean Beck Depression score for men was 12.8 while the mean for women was 15.4. Given the variability, the differences between men and women were not significantly different. Both men and women were approximately in the moderate range of depressive symptomatology (Beck, Ward, Mendelson, Mock, & Erbaugh, 1961; scores of 14 or greater). The impact ratings of psychological and physical aggression generally show that both can have a "quite negative" impact. Further, this research as well as that of others shows that the impact of psychological and physical aggression is not differential unless one is in a relationship that is characterized by being highly victimized.

Another way to assess the impact of psychological and physical aggression is to evaluate the impact of these variables on dropout from treatment (Brown, O'Leary, & Feldbau, 1997). In a treatment program designed to reduce both psychological and physical aggression, selection was made on the basis of husband and wife reports of husband-to-wife physical aggression. At least two incidents of physical aggression had to occur within the last year to be selected for a program comparing a gender-specific program with a couples program. In addition, the wives had to report in an individual assessment that they had not received injuries for which they sought medical attention and that they would not be fearful of participating with their husbands in treatment. There were positive changes reported by wives who completed the two different treatment programs, but there were no differential changes associated with the two treatments. More specifically, wives reported reductions in both psychological and physical aggression, increases in marital satisfaction, and decreases in anxiety and depression. However, 47% of the 70 couples dropped out of treatment. That is, they did not attend at least 10 of 14 treatment sessions (70% of the sessions). There was no difference in the dropout rates across the two treatments, and thus dropout results were assessed across the combined treatments. Demographic variables such as age, education, and income were not predictive of dropout. To our surprise, severity of physical aggression was not associated with dropout either. On the other hand, psychological aggression of the men and women was predictive of dropout.

Psychological aggression of the men as reported by the wives and as reflected on 14 items of the dominance/isolation scale of Tolman's Maltreatment of Women Scale was predictive of dropout. Psychological aggression of the women based on husband's reports on the six items of the psychological aggression measure from the Conflict Tactics Scale was predictive of dropout. Essentially, we interpreted these results as indicating that men's severe psychological aggression was predictive of dropout since the Tolman measure assesses dominance and control. While the men and women in the treatment program did not have significantly different scores on the dominance and control measure, the men had significantly higher scores on 4 of the 14 items, i.e., "my partner acted like I am his personal servant"; "my partner ordered me around"; "my partner didn't want me to go to school or other self-improvement activity"; and "my partner restricted my use of the telephone." There were no items on which the women had higher scores than men.

Mild psychological aggression as reported by husbands about the wives distinguished treatment completers from dropouts. Items on the psychological aggression scale of the CTS include: spouse insulted or swore at you; spouse refused to give sex or affection; spouse sulked and/or refused to talk about an issue; spouse stomped out of the room or house; spouse did or said something to spite you; and spouse threatened to leave the marriage. It is noteworthy that the mean level of husbands' mild psychological aggression was significantly higher than the wives' mild psychological aggression, but husbands' mild psychological aggression did not discriminate between completers and dropouts. It appears that when women engage in the above behaviors, they have a greater impact than when men engage in the same behaviors. Since men engaged in the behaviors more frequently than women, when women do display such psychological aggression, it may spell greater problems for the marriage in relationships characterized by considerable physical abuse. One reason for the greater predictability of dropout from treatment by psychological aggression of women (relative to physical aggression) may be that their physical aggression does not have as great a physical or psychological impact.

In a different research setting, batterers and their wives were followed over a 2 year period to assess predictors of marital dissolution (Jacobson, Gottman, Gortner, Berns, & Shortt, 1996). At the 2 year follow-up, 62% of the couples ($N = 24$) were still married while 38% ($N = 17$) had separated or divorced. Physical abuse did not discriminate between those relationships that terminated and those that did not. On the other hand, emotional abuse did. As they stated, "Over time, emotional abuse is a more important factor than physical abuse in contributing to wife's marital satisfaction, and in driving them out of the marriage."

The effects of psychological aggression are often intertwined with the effects of physical aggression (O'Leary & Jouriles, 1994), but the relative effects of psychological and physical aggression can be assessed in several ways. As was done by Folingstad and colleagues (1990), women who experience both types of aggression can rate the impact of them. One can assess depression, anxiety, fear, and self-esteem in women and men in relationships characterized by psychological aggression and those relationships characterized by both psychological and physical aggression. The other alternative, namely, physical aggression without psychological aggression is essentially nonexistent. More specifically, Stets showed that in a nationally representative sample, the Family Violence Survey of 1995, less than one half of one percent of individuals who are physically aggressive are not verbally aggressive. The effects of psychological and physical aggression can be examined indirectly by evaluating the different etiological paths leading to psychological and physical aggression in populations with (a) psychological aggression and (b) psychological and physical aggression. This approach has been used by Stets (1990) who found different patterns of relationships for the two groups. Using probit analyses in the National Family Violence Survey of 1985, she found that there were certain variables that were associated with using physical aggression that were not associated with verbal aggression alone, namely, women with a low occupation and income and men who approve of physical aggression. Stets' research provided support for the view that verbal and physical aggression are the result of a two-stage process with some factors being associated with physical aggression that are not associated with verbal aggression alone.

In populations where both psychological and physical aggression exist, the effects of psychological and physical aggression can be evaluated using various' methods, e.g., discriminant function analyses, regression, and path analytic models. Unfortunately, in studies of the effects of physical aggression, there are very few that provide data about the relative predictive power of psychological and physical aggression. However, as noted earlier (Brown, O'Leary, & Feldbau, 1997), in our sample of men and women seeking treatment for physical abuse, psychological aggression and physical aggression were used to predict dropout. Only psychological aggression predicted drop out. Clearly more studies assessing the relative contribution of psychological and physical aggression are needed. For example, in this miniseries, Arias and Pape (1999) demonstrated how psychological aggression had power in predicting a decision to leave a relationship that was over and above that of the physical aggression alone. In addition, in a sample of battered women either seeking shelter or nonshelter services, Sackett and Saunders (1999) found that fear was uniquely predicted by psychological abuse. Indeed, psychological abuse was a much stronger predictor of fear than physical abuse. Psychological abuse and physical abuse each contributed unique variance in depression and self-esteem. However, physical abuse accounted for more variance in depressive symptomatology than psychological abuse. In predicting self-esteem, both psychological and physical abuse made unique contributions, and they were of similar magnitude.

DEFINITION OF PSYCHOLOGICAL ABUSE IN INTIMATE RELATIONSHIPS

Adequate definitions of psychological abuse in relationships do not exist for legal and formal diagnostic purposes. The absence of such a definition, in part, reflects the greater emphasis on physical abuse of a partner by policy makers, mental health professionals, and by legal experts. The absence of such a definition also reflects the apparent ease of arriving at a definition of physical abuse of a partner because any act of physical aggression of a partner is often seen as partner abuse, particularly in divorce and custody matters. However, one must squarely address the very common prevalence of partner abuse in general populations of young married individuals that ranges from about 30%–35% of the men *and* women self-reporting such aggression (McLaughlin, Leonard, & Senchack, 1992; Mihalic, Elliot, & Menard, 1994; O'Leary et al., 1989). Moreover, physical aggression in the form of slapping, pushing, and shoving occurs in between 50% and 65% of the couples in marital clinic samples (cf. O'Leary, in press). Legal prosecution of everyone who hit a partner would be totally impractical as such prosecution, if totally effective, could involve arrest of one or both members of approximately half of all young married couples. Thus, it has become necessary to arrive at definitions of partner abuse for diagnostic purposes that involve more than a single instance of slapping or pushing (O'Leary & Jacobson, 1997).

While measures of psychological abuse exist that are reliable, the measures were not developed for legal purposes to help arrive at what would be an accepted definition of psychological abuse. Interestingly, however, neither were measures of physical abuse developed in order to arrive at what would be a DSM-IV type definition or a legal definition of abuse. Because of the prevalence of physical aggression by both men and women from adolescence to late adulthood (O'Leary & Cascardi, 1988), in DSM-IV, partner abuse has been defined as the presence of at least two acts of physical aggression within a year (or one severe act) and/or physical aggression that leads the partner to be fearful of the other or that results in injury requiring medical attention (O'Leary & Jacobson, 1997). Based on existing research, parallel definitions of psychological abuse lead to a definition as follows: acts of recurring criticism and/or verbal aggression toward a partner, and/or acts of isolation and domination of a partner. Generally, such actions cause the partner to be fearful of the other or lead the partner to have very low self-esteem, and it is recommended that researchers in this area routinely assess the impact of psychological abuse. Any definition of a problem or disorder can be altered as new evidence is gathered about a problem or disorder, as has been the case for numerous diagnostic classifications within the *Diagnostic and Statistical Manual* of the American Psychiatric Association. This will undoubtedly be the case for Physical Abuse of Partner and could be the case for Psychological Abuse of Partner.

SUMMARY

Psychological aggression has been measured reliably with at least eight different measures. The measures of psychological aggression can be differentiated from measures of physical aggression in factor analyses though there are consistently significant correlations between psychological and physical aggression. Psychological aggression generally precedes physical aggression. This adage is true both when one thinks about the development of relationships across time as well as when one thinks about the escalation of arguments in long-standing relationships. The evidence shows that psychological aggression predicts later physical aggression, and both are associated with deterioration in relationships. Data about the impact of psychological and physical aggression come from several quarters. Overall comparisons of physical and psychological aggression of women in physically abusive relationships indicated that the psychological abuse had a greater impact than the physical abuse. Direct impact ratings of psychological and physical aggression in both hypothetical and actual aggressive situations experienced by women in physically abusive relationships indicate that psychological aggression can have as negative an impact as physical aggression, unless a woman is in a highly victimized relationship. Associations of psychological aggression have been shown to be as great or greater with low self-esteem than with physical aggression. Further, psychological aggression predicted dropout from treatment and separation/divorce whereas physical aggression did not. Finally, major depressive episodes were more common where there were either threats of separation or actual separation/divorce or believing that an affair was ongoing than where physical aggression was seen by the wives as the severe negative marital event.

The data presented in this chapter in no way detract from the need to address issues of physical abuse. Rather, the data from a number of quarters indicate that psychological abuse can have a very negative impact and often one that is greater than physical abuse. As the impact of psychological aggression in relationships is accepted as having a role often as important as physical aggression, there will be greater attention to it. It is easier to have people from different professions such as law and mental health agree about what is physically abusive than what is psychologically aggressive, because there appears to be zero tolerance for physically abusive behaviors across disciplines. On the other hand, agreement about what level of psychological aggression would meet some legal or mental health criterion of psychological abuse seems harder because psychological aggression is so common, even in happily married couples. The ability to provide a readily acceptable definition of physical abuse may be illusory as it becomes evident that physical as well as psychological aggression is so common, particularly in young couples without marital discord (O'Leary & Cascardi, 1998). With such a realization, it may become evident that some judgment about the level of physical and psychological aggression, along with some impact ratings on the fear of the partner, may be necessary to move the field forward and to give the necessary significance to psychological aggression in a relationship and its adverse impact on the mental health of partners. Such an approach has been used with the diagnostic definition of physical abuse of partner (DSM-IV; O'Leary & Jacobson, 1997), and a parallel approach is offered herein as a practical means of having a definition of psychological abuse of partner.

REFERENCES

Aguilar, R. J., & Nightingale, N. N. (1994). The impact of specific battering experiences on the self-esteem of abused women. *Journal of Family Violence, 9,* 35-45.

Arias, I., & Pape, K. T. (1999). Psychological abuse: Implications for adjustment and commitment to leave violent partners. Article for miniseries on Psychological Abuse. *Violence and Victims, 14,* 55-67.

Beck, A., Ward, C., Mendelson, M., Mock, J., & Erbaugh, J. (1961). An inventory for measuring depression. *Archives of General Psychiatry, 4,* 561-571.

Brown, P. D., O'Leary, K. D., & Feldbau, S. R. (1997). Dropout in a treatment program for self-referring wife abusing men. *Journal of Family Violence, 12,* 365-387.

Berkowitz, L. (1973, July). The case for bottling up rage. *Psychology Today, 7,* 24-31.

Boyle, D., & Vivian, D. (1996). Generalized versus spouse-specific anger/hostility and men's violence against intimates. *Violence and Victims, 11,* 293-318.

Buss, A. H., & Durke, A. (1957). An inventory for assessing different kinds of hostility. *Journal of Consulting and Clinical Psychology, 21,* 343-349.

Campbell, D. W., Campbell, J., King, C., Parker, B., & Ryan, J. (1994). The reliability and factor structure of the index of spouse abuse with African American women. *Violence and Victims, 9,* 259-274.

Christian-Herman, J. L., O'Leary, K. D., & Avery-Leaf, S. (in press). The impact of severe negative marital events in marriage on depression. *Journal of Clinical Psychology.*

Deschner, J. P. (1984). *The hitting habit.* New York: The Free Press.

Eaton, W. W., Kramer, M., Anthony, J. C., Dryman, A., Shapiro, S., & Locke, B. Z. (1989). The incidence of specific DIS/DSM-II mental disorder: Data from the NIMH Epidemiological Catchment Area program. *Acta Psychiatrica Scandinavica, 79,* 163-178.

Folingstad, D. R., Rutledge, L. L., Berg, B. J., Hause, E. S., & Polek, D. S. (1990). The role of emotional abuse in physically abusive relationships. *Journal of Family Violence, 5,* 107-119.

Hamberger, L. K., & Hastings, J. E. (1986). Personality correlates of men who abuse their partners: A cross validation study. *Journal of Family Violence, 1,* 37-49.

Hamby, S. L. (1996). The dominance scale: Preliminary psychometric properties. *Violence and Victims, 11,* 199-212.

Holtzworth-Munroe, A., & Stuart, G. L. (1994). Topologies of male batterers: Three subtypes and the differences among them. *Psychological Bulletin, 116,* 476-497.

Hudson, W. W. (1990). *Partner abuse scale.* Tempe, AZ: Walmyr Publishing Company.

Hudson, W. W., & McIntosh, S. (1981). The index of spouse abuse. *Journal of Marriage and the Family, 43,* 873-888.

Jacobson, N. S., Gottman, J. M., Gortner, E., Berns, S., & Shortt, J. W. (1996). Psychological factors in the longitudinal course of battering: When do the couples split up? When does the abuse decrease? *Violence and Victims, 11,* 371-392.

Landau, P. (1976, May). A guide for the assertive book buyer. *Human Behavior, 70,* 64-71.

Lambert, L. K., & Fantuzzo, J. W. (1988). *Assessing spousal abuse: Beyond the Conflict Tactics Scales.* Unpublished master's thesis. California State University, Fullerton, CA.

Lawrence, E., & Bradbury, T. (1995). *Longitudinal course of physically aggressive and nonaggressive newlywed marriages.* Paper presented at the 29th annual meeting of the Association for Advancement of Behavior Therapy, Washington, DC.

McFarlane, J., Parker, B., Soeken, K., & Bullock, L. (1992). Assessing for abuse during pregnancy: Severity and frequency of injuries and associated entry into prenatal care. *Journal of the American Medical Association, 267*(23), 3176-3178.

McLaughlin, I. G., Leonard, K. E., & Senchak, M. (1992). Prevalence and distribution of premarital aggression among couples applying for a marriage license. *Journal of Family Violence, 7,* 309-319.

Marshall, L. L. (1992a). Development of the Severity of Violence Against Women Scales. *Journal of Family Violence, 7,* 103-121.

Marshall, L. L. (1992b). The Severity of Violence Against Men Scales. *Journal of Family Violence, 7,* 189-203.

Mihalic, S. W., Elliot, D. S., & Menard, S. (1994). Continuities in marital violence. *Journal of Family Violence, 9,* 195-225.

Murphy, C. M., & Cascardi, M. (1993). Psychological aggression and abuse in marriage. In R. L. Hampton, T. P. Gullotta, G. R. Adams, E. H. Potter, & R. P. Weissberg (Eds.), *Family violence: Prevention and treatment* (pp. 86-112). Sage: Newbury Park, CA.

Murphy, C., M., & O'Leary, K. D. (1989). Psychological aggression predicts physical aggression in early marriage. *Journal of Consulting and Clinical Psychology, 57,* 579-582.

O'Leary, K. D. (in press). Conjoint therapy for partners who engage in physically abusive behavior. *Journal of Aggression, Maltreatment, and Trauma.*

O'Leary, K. D. (1988). Physical aggression between spouses: A social learning perspective. In V. B. Van Hasselt, R. L. Morrison, A. S. Bellack, & M. Hersen (Eds.), *Handbook of family violence* (pp. 31-56). New York: Plenum.

O'Leary, K. D. (1993). Through a psychological lens: Personality traits, personality disorders, and levels of violence. In R. J. Gelles & D. R. Loseke (Eds.), *Current controversies on family violence* (pp. 7-29). Sage: Newbury Park, CA.

O'Leary, K. D., Barling, J., Arias, I. Rosenbaum, A., Malone, J., & Tyree, A. (1989). Prevalence and stability of physical aggression between spouses: A longitudinal analysis. *Journal of Consulting and Clinical Psychology, 57,* 263-268.

O'Leary, K. D., & Cascardi, M. (1998). Physical aggression in marriage: A developmental analysis. In T. N. Bradbury (Ed.), *The developmental course of marital dysfunction* (pp. 343-374). Cambridge, MA: Cambridge University Press.

O'Leary, K. D., & Curley, A. D. (1986). Assertion and family violence: Correlates of spouse abuse. *Journal of Marital and Family Therapy, 12*(3), 281-289.

O'Leary, K. D., Curley, A. D., Rosenbaum, A., & Clarke, C. (1985). Assertion training for abused wives: A potentially hazardous treatment. *Journal of Marital and Family Therapy, 11*(3), 319-322.

O'Leary, K. D., & Jacobson, N. S. (1997). Partner relational problems with physical abuse. *DSM IV Sourcebook* No. 4 (pp. 701-721). Washington, DC: American Psychiatric Press, Inc.

O'Leary, K. D., & Jouriles, E. N. (1994). Psychological abuse between adult partners: Prevalence and impact on partners and children. In L. L'Abate (Ed.), *Handbook of developmental family psychology and psychopathology* (pp. 330-349). New York: John Wiley & Sons.

O'Leary, K. D., Malone, J., & Tyree, A. (1994). Physical aggression in early marriage: Prerelationship and relationship effects. *Journal of Consulting and Clinical Psychology, 62,* 594-602.

Rathus, J. H., O'Leary, K. D., & Meyer, S. L. (1997). *Attachment, proximity control, and wife abuse.* Unpublished manuscript. University at Stony Brook, Stony Brook, NY.

Rhodes, N. R. (1985). *The assessment of psychological abuse: An alternative to the Conflict Tactics Scale.* Doctoral dissertation, Fuller Theological Seminary, 1985. Diss. Abstr. Int. 46: 2076B.

Rodenburg, F. A., & Fantuzzo, J. W. (1993). The measure of wife abuse: Steps toward the development of a comprehensive assessment technique. *Journal of Family Violence, 8,* 203-228.

Sackett, L. A., & Saunders, D. G. (1999). The impact of different forms of psychological abuse on battered women. Special Miniseries on Psychological Abuse. *Violence and Victims, 14,* 105-116.

Shepard, M. F., & Campbell, J. A. (1992). The abusive behavior inventory. *Journal of Interpersonal Violence, 7,* 291-305.

Stets, J. E. (1990). Verbal and physical aggression in marriage. *Journal of Marriage and the Family, 52,* 501-514.

Straus, M. A. (1979). Measuring intrafamily conflict and violence: The conflict tactics (CT) scales. *Journal of Marriage and the Family, 41,* 75-78.

Straus, M. A. (1994). Leveling, civility, and violence in the family. *Journal of Marriage and the Family, 35,* 13-29.

Straus, M. A., & Smith, C. (1990). Family patterns and child abuse. In M. A. Straus & R. J. Gelles (Eds.), *Physical violence in American families* (pp. 245-261). New Brunswick, NJ: Transaction Press.

Straus, M. A., Gelles, R. J., & Steinmetz, S. K. (1979). *Behind closed doors: Violence in the American family.* New York: Anchor/Doubleday.

Sullivan, C. M., Parisian, J. A., & Davidson, W. S. (1991, August). *Index of psychological abuse: Development of a measure.* Poster presentation at the annual conference of the American Psychological Association, San Francisco, CA.

Suitor, J. J., Pillemer, K., & Straus, M. A. (1990). In M. A. Straus & R. J. Gelles (Eds.), *Physical violence in American families* (pp. 305-317). New Brunswick, NJ: Transaction Press.

Straus, M. A., Hamby, S. L., Boney-McCoy, S., & Sugarman, D. (1995). The Revised Conflict Tactics Scales (CTS2). Durham, NH. Family Research Laboratory.

Tolman, R. M. (1989). The development of a measure of psychological maltreatment of women by their male partners. *Violence and Victims, 4,* 159-178.

Tolman, R. M. (1999). The validation of the psychological maltreatment of women inventory. *Violence and Victims, 14,* 25-37.

Vivian, D., & Langhinrichsen-Rohling, J. (1994). Are bi-directionally violent couples mutually victimized? A gender sensitive comparison. *Violence and Victims, 9,* 107-124.

Walker, L. E. (1979). *The battered woman.* New York: Harper & Row.

Chapter 2

Measuring Emotional Abuse in Dating Relationships as a Multifactorial Construct

Christopher M. Murphy and Sharon A. Hoover

Although a good deal of research has focused on physical aggression in dating relationships (e.g., Sugarman & Hotaling, 1989), very little work has examined emotional abuse in dating couples. This may be an unfortunate oversight given the apparent importance of emotional abuse in the development of physical relationship aggression. Longitudinal studies of newlywed couples, for example, have demonstrated that psychological aggression predicts the initiation and frequency of physical aggression (Leonard & Senchak, 1996; Murphy & O'Leary, 1989; O'Leary, Malone, & Tyree, 1994). At the severe end of the spectrum, the vast majority of clinical spouse batterers display a pervasive pattern of emotional abuse that occurs more frequently than physical violence (Murphy & Cascardi,1999). In addition to its apparent role in the development of physical abuse, emotional abuse can exert very negative effects. Over 70% of formerly battered women, for example, report that emotional abuse had more profound negative effects than physical abuse (Follingstad, Rutledge, Berg, Hause, & Polek, 1990).

Further research on emotional abuse in dating relationships may have a number of important implications. Such work may elucidate developmental processes associated with relationship violence. Emotional abuse may also prove useful in detecting individuals and couples at high risk for physical aggression. Research on emotional abuse may enhance our understanding of the consequences of abuse in dating relationships, including the ways in which abuse experiences may influence the development of intimate relationships and the capacity for intimacy.

Although there is no widely accepted definition of psychological or emotional abuse, some key elements appear consistently in working definitions of this construct. Murphy and Cascardi (1999) suggest that psychological abuse "consists of coercive or aversive acts intended to produce emotional harm or threat of harm." Unlike physically abusive behaviors, which are directed at the target's bodily integrity, psychologically abusive behaviors are directed at the target's emotional well-being or sense of self. Psychologically abusive behaviors often produce fear, increase dependency, or damage the self-concept of the recipient. This working definition characterizes a wide range of intimate relationship behaviors, spanning the continuum from mildly coercive actions that occur occasionally in well-adjusted relationships to a comprehensive pattern of coercive domination and mind control found in the most extreme battering relationships (Graham, Rawlings, & Rimini, 1988; Romero, 1985).

Assessment issues remain a critical priority for advances in this area. Existing measures contain brief lists of aggressive acts, mostly verbal in nature (e.g., Hudson & McIntosh, 1981; O'Leary & Curley, 1986; Straus, 1979; Straus, Hamby, Boney-McCoy, & Sugarman, 1996), or lengthy lists of highly coercive behaviors designed to characterize long-term, severe battering relationships (e.g., Tolman, 1989). At the empirical level, many questions remain about whether these measures adequately assess the broad domain of emotional abuse as defined above. Clinical and qualitative investigations of battered women and women in distressed relationships have identified several subcategories of abusive behaviors, such as isolating and restricting the partner's activities and social contacts, attacking the partner's self-esteem through humiliating and degrading comments, withdrawing in hostile ways, destroying property, and threatening harm or violence (Murphy & Cascardi, 1999). Yet the existing measures do not appear to assess these different aspects of psychological abuse as distinct factors.

Factor analyses of measures with a small number of psychological aggression items, such as Straus's Conflict Tactics Scale (1979), identify psychological aggression as a single, unidimensional factor that is distinct from physical aggression (e.g., Barling, O'Leary, Jouriles, Vivian, & MacEwen, 1987; Straus, 1979). Factor analyses of more involved measures generally fail to support complex hypothesized factor structures, and provide factors that are difficult to interpret in light of the clinical and qualitative studies. In developing the Psychological Maltreatment of Women Inventory (PMWI), for example, Tolman (1989) originally identified 6 conceptually distinct forms of psychological abuse, yet the factor analysis revealed only 2 factors, each a complex amalgam of topographically diverse abusive behaviors. As yet, there is relatively little evidence that the two factors of the PMWI have discriminant validity.

More recently, multiple, coherent factors have emerged from factor analyses of item severity ratings in measures of abusive behavior (Marshall, 1992; Rodenburg & Fantuzzo, 1993). Item severity ratings reflect the perceived severity or impact of various abusive behaviors, but do not necessarily reflect patterning in the perpetration of abusive behavior (e.g., Marshall, 1992; Rodenburg & Fantuzzo, 1993). Marshall (1992), for example, asked a large sample of college students to provide hypothetical ratings of how serious, aggressive, abusive, threatening, and violent each of 49 abusive acts would be if a man did them to a woman. Symbolic acts, threats, physical violence, and sexual violence emerged from factor analysis of these item severity ratings. It is important to note, however, that distinct and coherent patterns of perceived item severity from hypothetical ratings may not adequately characterize behavioral patterns that are organized around similarities in behavioral topography or function.

Marshall (1996) subsequently used cluster analysis to examine more specific patterns of psychological abuse victimization. On the basis of 51 psychological abuse items, she identified 6 clusters of women from a large sample who had experienced relationship distress. This work identified items that were relatively high, moderate, or low in endorsement frequency for each cluster of subjects. The clusters differed somewhat in the patterning of behaviors characterized as isolation, dominance, control, withdrawal, and criticism. The overall levels of psychological abuse exposure, exposure to violent threats, and violent victimization also varied among clusters. Although the clusters of abuse victims were not given specific labels or precise definitions, this study was unique in providing empirical support for the idea that there are distinct patterns of psychological abuse victimization. Because individuals, rather than behaviors or items, were clustered, however, the results did not clearly identify how different abusive behaviors covary. Thus, the study demonstrated that there are different clusters of emotional abuse victims, but it did not provide a method for grouping abusive behaviors into coherent clusters or patterns.

The goal of the current research was to explore the feasibility and utility of assessing emotional abuse as a multifactorial construct using a priori definitions of different forms of emotional abuse. This work represents an initial step in the development and validation of a multifactorial measure of emotional abuse in dating relationships. It began with a systematic review of the literature on psychological abuse in marriage and dating relationships (Murphy &

Cascardi, 1999), which identified common forms of emotional abuse. Next, potential items were selected from several sources to represent the domain of emotional abuse. Items were rewritten if necessary for clarity and applicability to dating relationships, and additional items were generated to apply to the dating context. Items to assess economic abuse were excluded because most dating couples maintain separate finances. Items to assess male privilege were excluded because most refer to cohabitating relationships or to the behavior of only one gender, potentially limiting the applicability to dating or same-sex relationships. Items to assess minimization and denial of physical abuse effects were also excluded as these behaviors are relevant only to physically violent relationships.

Further review of item content and recent literature suggested a 4-factor model. The factors were based on the form of the behaviors expressed and presumptions about their intended emotional consequences. First, threats, property violence, and intense displays of verbal aggression were lumped together into a category labeled *Dominance / Intimidation,* under the assumption that the intended effect of these behaviors is to produce fear or submission through the display of aggression. Second, behaviors intended to isolate the partner and restrict the partner's activities and social contacts, along with intense displays of jealousy and possessiveness, were lumped together under the assumption that their intended effect is to limit perceived threats to the relationship by increasing the partner's dependency and availability. Originally labeled "proximity maintenance," following Rathus (1994), this category was relabeled *Restrictive Engulfment* to capture the coercive nature of these behaviors. Third, humiliating and degrading behaviors were lumped into a category labeled *Denigration,* under the assumption that their main intended effect is to reduce, through direct attacks, the partner's self-esteem. Fourth, the tendency to withhold emotional contact and withdraw from the partner in a hostile fashion was included in a category labeled *Hostile Withdrawal,* under the assumption that these behaviors are intended to punish the partner and increase the partner's anxiety or insecurity about the relationship. Similar forms of abuse have been elucidated by clinicians and qualitative researchers (see reviews by Marshall, 1994; Murphy & Cascardi,1999).

This chapter describes two preliminary investigations of two female college dating samples using a provisional, 54-item measure designed to assess these 4 hypothesized forms of emotional abuse. The working hypothesis was that these 4 forms of abuse would constitute coherent behavioral patterns as indicated by factor analysis, and that they would have somewhat different associations with physical dating aggression and with other aspects of interpersonal functioning. Scale development was conceived of as an iterative process. The first step was to explore empirically whether it would be feasible and useful to measure emotional abuse in dating relationships as a multifactorial construct using the 4-factor model described above. If this model were empirically validated, then future studies could be designed to refine the item set used to assess these patterns of abuse, to validate their different hypothesized interpersonal functions, to explore developmental histories that may be associated with these distinct forms of emotional abuse, and to explore their implications for the development of physical relationship violence and severe battering relationships

METHODS

Participants

All study participants were in current dating relationships and had never been previously married. Participants received course credit in introductory psychology for participating. Sample 1 was obtained during the 1995–96 academic year and consisted of 71 females. Their average age was 20.1 (SD = 2.2). Regarding racial and ethnic background, 21% were African American, 10% were Asian American, 59% were Caucasian, and 4% were of other racial or ethnic origins. The mean length of dating relationship was 18.5 months (median = 12; SD = 15.0); 11.3% were cohabiting with their partners at the time of the study. Sample 2 was obtained during the 1996–97 academic year and consisted of 86 females. Their average age was 19.1 (SD = 1.9). Regarding racial and ethnic background, 21% were African American, 20% were Asian American, 1% were Hispanic, 45% were Caucasian, and 5% were of other racial or ethnic origins. The mean length of dating relationship was 16.2 months (median = 11; SD = 16.1); 7% were cohabiting with their partners at the time of the study.

Measures

Emotional Abuse Scale Development. In prior work, an initial 34-item set with data from 160 students in dating relationships was used to construct preliminary scales for the four subtypes of abuse.[1] Items were subsequently discarded if they had low response frequencies (fewer than 10% of individuals reporting any occurrence by self or partner), item-scale correlations less than .25, or poor differential correlation (difference between corrected item-scale correlation and the correlation with any of the other three scales < .1). New items were generated based on the first author's clinical experience with domestic abuse perpetrators and by a group of undergraduate research assistants who engaged in informal discussions with friends and acquaintances in dating relationships about the four types of behavior included in the assessment. Some items were rewritten to clarify meaning, and the response format was simplified. Participants were asked to report how often they themselves and their dating partner performed each behavior in the past 4 months on a 7-point frequency scale (never, once, twice, 3–5 times, 6–10 times,

11–20 times, and more than 20 times). The result was a revised, 54-item set with 4 subscales derived on a rational, a priori basis. Example items for each subscale are listed in Table 1. The internal consistency (coefficient alpha) of the four rationally derived subscales in the combined sample for reports of abusive behaviors by self and partner, respectively, were .84 and . 85 for Restrictive Engulfment (13 items), .88 and .91 for Hostile Withdrawal (9 items), .89 and .92 for Denigration (17 items), and .83 and .91 for Domination / Intimidation (15 items).

Physical Aggression was assessed with the eight physical aggression items of the Conflict Tactics Scale (CTS), a widely used and face-valid measure of adult relationship aggression that has been used in national survey studies, has adequate internal consistency, and has shown significant correlations with a number of hypothesized correlates of relationship violence (Straus, 1979; 1990). The assessment time frame was adapted for the current study to be consistent with the emotional abuse measure. Participants reported on the frequency of their own and their partner's aggression during the 4 months prior to the assessment.

Social Desirability Response Bias was assessed with the 40-item Balanced Inventory of Desirable Responding- Version 6 (BIDR-6; Paulhus, 1991). The BIDR consists of two factor-analytically derived subscales. One subscale measures Self-

**Table 1. Highest Loading Items From the Rotated Solution
on the Four Factors of Emotional Abuse**

Factor 1: Hostile Withdrawal
  Sulked or refused to talk about issue
  Refused to acknowledge problem
  Refused to discuss problem
  Acted cold or distant when angry
Factor 2: Domination/Intimidation
Told "you'll never get away from me" in an angry or threatening way[a]
  Threatened to throw something at partner
  Intentionally destroyed belongings
  Threatened to harm partner's friends
Factor 3: Denigration
  Said that partner would never amount to anything
  Called partner a loser, failure, or similar term
  Called partner ugly
  Called partner worthless
Factor 4: Restrictive Engulfment
  Complained partner spends too much time w/ friends
  Asked where s/he had been or who s/he had been with in a suspicious manner
  Got angry because partner went somewhere w/o telling him/her
  Tried to make partner feel guilty for not spending time together

[a]Item assigned a priori to Restrictive Engulfment subscale.
Note. Copies of the complete item wordings and scale instructions are available upon request from the first author.

Deception (*SD*), the tendency to provide honestly held but inflated descriptions of the self. The other subscale measures Impression Management (IM), the tendency to dissimulate by providing inflated self-descriptions in public settings. Available evidence suggests that self-reports of emotional abuse by batterers are significantly and negatively correlated with both self-deception and impression management on the BIDR, whereas self-reports of physical abuse are significantly correlated only with the impression management scale (Dutton & Hemphill, 1992).

Interpersonal Problems were assessed with the circumplex scales of the Inventory of Interpersonal Problems (IIP; Alden, Wiggins, & Pincus, 1990; Horowitz, Rosenberg, Baer, Ureno, & Villasenor, 1988). The eight circumplex scales utilize 64 of the original 127 IIP items, and measure interpersonal difficulties labeled Domineering, Intrusive, Overly Nurturant, Exploitable, Nonassertive, Socially Avoidant, Cold, and Vindictive. The 64 items were selected empirically to best represent a circumplex structure for the scale. Participants report on a 5-point Likert scale the degree to which specific interpersonal problems apply to themselves. In a large validation sample, the scales had adequate internal consistency (.7 and above) and demonstrated the predicted pattern of validity correlations with the interpersonal circumplex as assessed by Wiggins' Revised Interpersonal Adjective Scale (Alden et al., 1990; Wiggins, Trapnell, & Phillips, 1988). The interpersonal problem circumplex has been used to validate measures of interpersonal functioning by locating them in the circumplex through trigonometric procedures. These methods can be used to investigate the specific nature of interpersonal problem measurement instruments in light of the structural criterion imposed by the interpersonal circumplex (Gurtman, 1992).

Attachment was assessed with subscales from the Reciprocal Attachment Questionnaire (West & Sheldon-Keller, 1994). Subscales were chosen for the current investigation to assess problematic attachment qualities that are not overlapping in content with the emotional abuse scales. Three attachment dimension subscales, assessing proximity seeking, separation protest, and feared loss, contain three items each. Subscales for the attachment patterns of compulsive care giving, compulsive self-reliance, and compulsive care-seeking contain seven items each. Participants rate the degree to which each item is descriptive of them on a 5-point scale. The subscales were theoretically derived, and had adequate internal consistency (above .7) in the development sample.

Procedures

Participants completed questionnaires in classrooms in groups of 8–15. All participants completed the emotional abuse items, physical abuse scale, and social desirability measure. Sample 2 participants also completed the interpersonal problem and attachment measures.

RESULTS

Principle Components Analysis. A principle components analysis (PCA) with varimax rotation was used to explore the factor structure of the 54-item set using data from females in both samples ($N = 157$). One item was deleted because there was no variance (i.e., no one reported that this behavior had occurred). Because reports of abuse by the self may be more biased by social desirability and may contain less variance than reports of abuse by the partner (Arias & Beach, 1987; Dutton & Hemphill, 1992; Riggs, Murphy, & O'Leary, 1989), the PCA was conducted only on the female participants' reports of their partners' abusive behaviors.

The PCA yielded 12 factors with eigen values greater than 1. Visual analysis of the scree plot suggested a 4-factor solution. Three and five factor solutions were also examined but were not readily interpretable. The first 4 factors accounted cumulatively for 55% of the variance in the set of 53 items. Table 1 contains example items with the highest loadings on each of the 4 factors. The solution in general conformed to the predicted 4-factor model. The highest loading items on each of the 4 rotated factors correspond to the conceptually derived subscales for Hostile Withdrawal, Domination/Intimidation, Denigration, and Restrictive Engulfment, respectively. Of the 53 items, 39 had their highest loadings on the predicted factor. Of the remaining 14 items, 5 also had secondary loadings above .3 on the predicted factor. Given (a) that the 4-factor solution corresponded quite well to the original model, (b) that sampling error can effect factor loadings, and (c) that only data from females were analyzed, the decision was made to retain the original, rationally derived item assignments in computing subscale scores rather than to reassign or delete items based on the factor analysis. Further efforts are under-way to explore the factor structure of this item set with male subjects, to produce a smaller set of items that are univocal with respect to these four factors, and to conduct a confirmatory analysis of the 4-factor solution. Nonetheless, the current results support the provisional use of the four rationally derived subscales in order to explore differential associations with other variables.

Associations with Physical Aggression. Table 2 displays the product-moment correlations between the four rationally derived subscales of emotional abuse and the CTS physical aggression scale. As expected from prior studies of psychological and physical abuse (e.g., Murphy & O'Leary, 1989; Straus, 1974), all of the

Table 2. Correlations with Physical Aggression ($N = 157$)

Emotional Abuse Subscale	Abuse by Partner	Abuse by Self
Restrictive Engulfment	.45**	.46**
Hostile Withdrawal	.46**	.29**
Denigration	.72**	.56**
Dominance/Intimidation	.74**	.67**

**p < .01.

correlations were significant. There were differences, however, in the strength of association between the different emotional abuse subscales and physical aggression. The physical aggression associations for Denigration and Dominance/Intimidation were higher than the associations for Restrictive Engulfment and Hostile Withdrawal.

Statistical tests were conducted to determine whether these correlations differed significantly in magnitude (Snedecor & Cochran, 1980, pp. 186–187). For reports of abusive behavior by one's partner, an omnibus test revealed a significant difference in the magnitude of the four emotional abuse subscale correlations with physical aggression (chi-squared = 29.47, df = 3, p < .01). The physical aggression correlations with Denigration and Dominance/Intimidation were each significantly higher (p < .01) than the physical aggression correlations with Restrictive Engulfment and Hostile Withdrawal. For reports of abusive behavior by one's self, an omnibus test again revealed significant differences in the magnitude of correlations with physical aggression (chi-squared = 21.6, df = 3, p < .01). The physical aggression correlation with Dominance/Intimidation was significantly higher (p < .01) than the physical aggression correlations with both Hostile Withdrawal and Restrictive Engulfment. The physical aggression correlation with Denigration was significantly higher (p < .01) than the correlation with Hostile Withdrawal, but not significantly different from the correlation with Restrictive Engulfment. In summary, although all four forms of emotional abuse were significantly associated with physical aggression, two forms of abuse, Denigration and Dominance / Intimidation, had stronger associations with physical aggression than did Hostile Withdrawal and Restrictive Engulfment.

Associations With Social Desirability. Table 3 presents the emotional abuse subscale correlations with social desirability. All of the correlations were in the expected direction, with those who scored higher on the social desirability scales

Table 3. Correlations With Social Desirability (N = 157)

Emotional Abuse Subscale	Abuse by Self		Abuse by Partner	
	Impression Management	Self-Deception	Impression Management	Self-Deception
Restrictive Engulfment	-.26**	-.23**	-.07ns	-.02ns
Hostile Withdrawal	-.22**	-.11ns	-.30**	-.17*
Denigration	-.24**	-.14ns	-.12ns	-.11ns
Dominance/ Intimidation	-.24**	-.13ns	-.12ns	-.07ns
Physical Aggression	-.15ns	-.09ns	-.08ns	-.03ns

ns = non significant. *p < .05. **p < .01.

reporting less abusive behavior. Reports of abuse by self on all four subscales were significantly associated with Impression Management. Only the Restrictive Engulfment subscale for reports of abuse by self was significantly associated with Self-Deception. For abuse by the partner, the Hostile Withdrawal subscale was significantly associated with both Impression Management and Self-Deception, whereas the other abuse subscales were not significantly associated with social desirability. It appears that conscious impression management may have a consistent, modest influence on self-reports of emotional abuse. The Impression Management component of social desirability was more consistently associated with abuse reports than was the Self-Deception component. Finally, as would be expected from past studies (e.g., Arias & Beach, 1987; Dutton & Hemphill, 1992), reports of abuse by the self were more consistently associated with social desirability than were reports of abuse by the partner.

Associations with Interpersonal Problems. Table 4 contains correlations with the circumplex scales of the Inventory of Interpersonal Problems (IIP). The four emotional abuse subscales had some common associations with the broader domain of interpersonal problems. All of the subscales were significantly associated with the Domineering, Vindictive, and Intrusive scales of the IIP. None of the abuse subscales was significantly associated with the Overly Nurturant, Exploitable, Nonassertive, and Socially Avoidant scales of the IIP. Thus, the emotional abuse scales clearly covaried with interpersonal problems associated with control rather than passivity.

Trigonometric procedures were used to locate the subscales within the circumplex by calculating coordinates along the X axis (nurturance) and Y axis (dominance) based on linear composites of scale correlations calculated through cosine and sine weightings, respectively, of the theoretical angular locations of the 8 circumplex scales (Gurtman, 1992; Wiggins, Phillips, & Trapnell, 1989). The subscale loca-

Table 4. Correlations With the Circumplex Scales of the Inventory of Interpersonal Problems ($N = 86$)

	Emotional Abuse Subscale (Abuse by Self)			
IIP Scale	Restrictive Engulfment	Hostile Withdrawal	Denigration	Dominance/ Intimidation
Cold	.05*ns*	.27*	.17*ns*	.11*ns*
Vindictive	.36**	.38**	.37**	.41**
Domineering	.37**	.34**	.39**	.30**
Intrusive	.40**	.25*	.31**	.28*
Overly Nurturant	.19*ns*	-.04*ns*	.04*ns*	.08*ns*
Exploitable	.19*ns*	.04*ns*	.08*ns*	-.02*ns*
Nonassertive	.16*ns*	.13*ns*	.17*ns*	.05*ns*
Socially Avoidant	.15*ns*	.14*ns*	.16*ns*	.03*ns*

ns = non significant. *$p < .05$. **$p < .01$.

tions are depicted in Figure 1. All of the subscales were located in the top half of the circumplex, in proximity to the Domineering octant, suggesting convergent validity with regard to problems controlling, manipulating, and aggressing toward others (Alden et al., 1990). Dominance / Intimidation, in particular, was located quite specifically within the Domineering octant (angular location = 102°). Restrictive Engulfment was located half way between the Domineering and Intrusive octants (angular location = 69°), indicating an association with problems involving inappropriate self-disclosure, attention seeking, and difficulty being alone (Alden et al., 1990). Denigration was located on the other side of the Domineering octant, half way to the Vindictive octant (angular location = 114°), and Hostile Withdrawal was located within the Vindictive octant (angular location = 132°). These locations indicate an association with problems involving suspiciousness, distrust, and insensitivity.

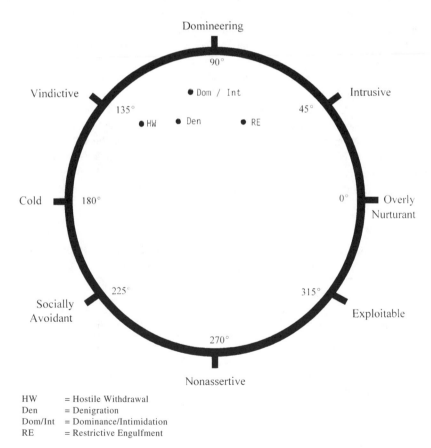

HW   = Hostile Withdrawal
Den   = Denigration
Dom/Int = Dominance/Intimidation
RE   = Restrictive Engulfment

Figure 1. Inventory of Interpersonal Problems Circumplex

In general, it appears that all four emotional abuse subscales converge in measuring behaviors that are linked to problems with dominance, coercion, and aggression. The subscales vary, however, along the affiliative dimension of the interpersonal problem circumplex, ranging from hyper-affiliative forms of coercion, such as Restrictive Engulfment, to nonaffiliative forms of coercion such as Hostile Withdrawal. These results again suggest that it may be useful to discriminate among patterns of emotional abuse, which have overlapping, yet somewhat discernable, associations with the broader domain of interpersonal problems.

Associations With Attachment Variables. Table 5 displays associations between reports of abuse by the self and selected RAQ subscales. The first three attachment scales measure qualities, which, when strongly endorsed, are associated with anxious/insecure attachment (separation protest, proximity seeking, and feared loss). Restrictive Engulfment had substantial associations with all three of these attachment subscales. Separation Protest also had significant, yet modest, correlations with the three other forms of emotional abuse. These results suggest that anxious preoccupation with attachment concerns, although somewhat associated with all four forms of emotional abuse, were most strongly and most consistently associated with Restrictive Engulfment.

The last three attachment scales in Table 5 measure strategies for regulating closeness and related emotions. None of the abuse subscales was significantly associated with Compulsive Care Giving or Compulsive Self-reliance. This finding is consistent with the lack of significant associations with the Overly Nurturant, Exploitable, Nonassertive, and Socially Avoidant scales of the IIP. Restrictive Engulfment, Hostile Withdrawal, and Denigration were all significantly associated with Compulsive Care-seeking, further indicating, at least for the female sample investigated, that attachment concerns are associated with emotionally abusive behaviors.

Table 5. Correlations With Select Subscales From the Reciprocal Attachment Questionnaire (*N* = 86)

IIP Scale	Restrictive Engulfment	Hostile Withdrawal	Denigration	Dominance/ Intimidation
	Emotional Abuse Subscale (Abuse by Self)			
Proximity Seeking	.34**	.12ns	.19ns	.12ns
Separation Protest	.52**	.28*	.25*	.26*
Feared Loss	.38**	.17ns	.18ns	.18ns
Compulsive Care-Giving	.14ns	.00ns	-.04ns	.09ns
Compulsive Care Seeking	.33**	.29**	.24*	.22ns
Compulsive Self Reliance	-.03ns	.17ns	.10ns	.05ns

ns = non significant. *p < .05. **p < .01.

DISCUSSION

The major goal of the investigation was to explore the feasibility and utility of assessing emotional abuse in dating relationships as a multifactorial construct. The alternative approaches are to measure emotional abuse as a unidimensional construct, or to make distinctions based on severity, but not based on the form or intended consequences of emotionally abusive behavior. An exploratory principle components analysis supported the hypothesized 4-factor model of emotional abuse. Distinct dimensions were uncovered that corresponded to the descriptive behavioral categories of Restrictive Engulfment, Hostile Withdrawal, Denigration, and Dominance / Intimidation. The potential utility of assessing these factors as separate variables was apparent in differential correlations with physical aggression and the broad domain of interpersonal problems.

The following is a brief synopsis of the four types of abuse based on the current findings. *Restrictive Engulfment* involves tracking, monitoring, and controlling the partner's activities and social contacts, along with efforts to squelch perceived threats to the relationship. This behavior pattern was consistently associated with signs of anxious and insecure attachment and a compulsive need for nurturance. In a prior study with an earlier emotional abuse item set, this pattern was highly associated with interpersonal dependency, relationship-specific dependency, jealousy, and other dependency-related variables (Murphy, Hartman, Muccino, & Douchis, 1995). Intrusiveness is apparent as an associated interpersonal problem but coldness is not. Restrictive engulfment has a moderate association with physical aggression, suggesting that it is somewhat independent of physical abuse in dating relationships.

Hostile Withdrawal involves avoidance of the partner during conflict and withholding of emotional availability or contact with the partner in a cold or punitive fashion. Hostile Withdrawal was associated with a range of interpersonal problems that included being cold, vindictive, and domineering. It had a moderate association with one aspect of attachment anxiety, namely, separation protest. Hostile Withdrawal had a low to moderate association with physical aggression. It is possible that affective disengagement during conflict may serve a protective function against escalation to physical aggression for some individuals, an idea that was used in other research to explain why nonviolent men in discordant relationships appear to be less emotionally invested in their relationships when compared to both happily married men and domestically violent men (Murphy, Meyer, & O'Leary, 1994).

Denigration involves humiliating and degrading attacks on the partner's self-esteem. This behavior pattern had a moderate to strong correlation with physical aggression and a moderate correlation with attachment insecurities, namely, separation protest and compulsive care-seeking. With regard to the circumplex of interpersonal problems, Denigration was primarily associated with being vindictive and domineering.

Dominance / Intimidation involves threats, property violence, and intense verbal aggression. Of the four emotional abuse patterns, this one has the most overt similarity to physical aggression. Not surprisingly, Dominance / Intimidation was highly correlated with physical aggression. This pattern had a moderate, significant association with attachment insecurities in the form of separation protest. Its association with the circumplex of interpersonal problems was fairly specific to the domineering region of the circumplex. Although Denigration and Dominance / Intimidation had quite similar associations with interpersonal problems and physical aggression, the factor analysis results suggest that they are distinct forms of emotional abuse.

One of the most important questions in research on adult relationship abuse is how these patterns develop in the life-span of individuals and in the course of specific relationships (O'Leary & Cascardi, 1998). The current results suggest, not surprisingly, that an aggressive, vindictive, and controlling interpersonal style is important to emotionally abusive behavior in general. The results also implicate attachment insecurities, and problems being insensitive and cold, as important correlates of specific forms of emotional abuse. It appears that the different forms of emotional abuse may have both shared and unique origins in personality and social development. The interpersonal characteristics associated with abusive behavior may also influence assortative partner selection and the development, maintenance, and dissolution of dating relationships.

Prior clinical and qualitative work, in general, has conceptualized emotional abuse in light of the comprehensive pattern of coercive domination that often characterizes severe spouse batterers. The finding that Dominance/Intimidation and Denigration were very highly related to physical aggression supports the strong theoretical connection between physical and psychological aggression. This finding also implies that many of the prior measures of psychological aggression, such as the CTS, which contain items that would fall primarily on these two factors, have assessed quite central and important aspects of psychological abuse.

The current 4-factor model raises the additional possibility that some people in the general population will experience specific patterns, such as Hostile Withdrawal and Restrictive Engulfment, that although quite distressing, are topographically dissimilar to physical relationship aggression and may occur in the absence of physical aggression. Further analysis of such patterns may be helpful in broadening our understanding of coercive and abusive relationship behaviors, and may also prove helpful in efforts to detect less intense forms of emotional abuse for prevention and early intervention programs focused on the development of healthy relationships.

Social desirability, in the form of conscious impression management, had a modest, consistent influence on reports of one's own emotionally abusive behavior, and a less consistent influence on reports of the partner's abusive behavior. The magnitude and pattern of social desirability correlations are consistent with the conclusion of a recent meta-analysis by Sugarman and

Hotaling (1997), which reported a weighted average social desirability correlation with physical relationship aggression of -.18. The current results provided only limited and inconsistent support for the idea that emotional abuse reports are associated with the self-deception component of social desirability as well as impression management component, as reported by Dutton and Hemphill (1992). Self-deception was associated with self-reports of Restrictive Engulfment, but not with the other forms of emotional abuse. It is possible that self-enhancement processes specifically contaminate reports of Restrictive Engulfment behaviors involving efforts to monitor, track, and maintain proximity to the partner through coercive means. Self-enhancing rationalizations may lead to the belief that these behaviors were in the best interests of the partner or the relationship, therefore limiting reports in the context of an inventory containing obviously abusive or harmful behaviors.

Although the current findings suggest that it is feasible and potentially useful to conceptualize and measure emotional abuse in dating relationships as a multifactorial construct, further work is ongoing to validate and extend the multifactorial model. Gender differences in correlations with interpersonal problems and attachment qualities were not examined in the current study. Although there are few compelling reasons at the present time to expect gender differences in the developmental and personality correlates of emotional abuse, this remains an important topic for further investigation. In addition, the current investigation of college students may not generalize to less academically talented samples or to other age groups. Finally, the correlational analyses used rationally derived subscales of emotional abuse which were only partially supported by the factor analysis. Future work with larger samples will be necessary to refine the subscales based on empirical findings, and to finalize a version of this measure that contains clear factors within a confirmatory model with a smaller set of items that are univocal with respect to the factors.

In summary, the results provide support for the feasibility and utility of assessing psychological abuse in dating relationships as a multifactorial construct, with four distinct forms of emotional abuse . All four forms of emotional abuse converged in being associated with interpersonal problems related to control, manipulation, and aggressiveness. Two specific forms of emotional abuse, Dominance/Intimidation and Denigration, were very strongly associated with physical relationship aggression. Two other forms, Hostile Withdrawal and Restrictive Engulfment, had more modest associations with physical aggression, and were quite distinct in their location along the affiliative dimension of the interpersonal problem circumplex. Restrictive Engulfment had the most consistent and strongest associations with self-reported attachment insecurities. This work represents an initial step in modeling different forms of emotionally abusive behavior that may eventually prove useful in understanding the development of adult relationship dysfunction and domestic violence.

REFERENCES

Alden, L. E., Wiggins J. S., & Pincus, A. L. (1990). Construction of circumplex scales for the Inventory of Interpersonal Problems. *Journal of Personality Assessment, 55,* 521-536.

Arias, I., & Beach, S. R. H. (1987). Validity of self-reports of marital violence. *Journal of Family Violence, 2,* 139-149.

Barling, J., O'Leary, K. D., Jouriles, E. N., Vivian, D., & MacEwen, K. E. (1987). Factor similarity of the Conflict Tactics Scales across samples, spouses, and sites: Issues and implications. *Journal of Family Violence, 2,* 37-54.

Dutton, D. G., & Hemphill, K. J. (1992). Patterns of socially desirable responding among perpetrators and victims of wife assault. *Violence and Victims, 7,* 29-39.

Follingstad, D. R., Rutledge, L. L., Berg, B. J., Hause, E. S., & Polek, D. S. (1990). The role of emotional abuse in physically abusive relationships. *Journal of Family Violence, 5,* 107-120.

Graham, D. L. R., Rawlings, E., & Rimini, N. (1988). Survivors of terror: Battered women, hostages and the Stockholm Syndrome. In K. Yllo & M. Bograd (Eds.), *Feminist perspectives on wife abuse* (pp. 217-233). Beverly Hills, CA: Sage.

Gurtman, M. B. (1992). Construct validity of interpersonal personality measures: The interpersonal circumplex as a nomological net. *Journal of Personality and Social Psychology, 63,* 105-118.

Horowitz, L. M., Rosenberg, S. E., Baer, B. A., Ureno, G., & Villasenor, V. S. (1988). Inventory of Interpersonal Problems: Psychometric properties and clinical applications. *Journal of Consulting and Clinical Psychology, 56,* 885-892.

Hudson, W. W., & McIntosh, S. R. (1981). The assessment of spouse abuse: Two quantifiable dimensions. *Journal of Marriage and the Family, 43,* 873-888.

Leonard, K. E., & Senchak, M. (1996). Prospective prediction of husband marital aggression within newlywed couples. *Journal of Abnormal Psychology, 105,* 368-380.

Marshall, L. L. (1992). Development of the Severity of Violence Against Women Scales. *Journal of Family Violence, 7,* 103-121.

Marshall, L. L. (1994). Physical and psychological abuse. In W. R. Cupach & B. H. Spitzberg (Eds.), *The dark side of interpersonal communication* (pp. 281-311). Hillsdale, NJ: Lawrence Erlbaum.

Marshall, L. L. (1996). Psychological abuse of women: Six distinct clusters. *Journal of Family Violence, 11,* 369-399.

Murphy, C. M., & Cascardi, M. (1999). Psychological abuse in marriage and dating relationships. In R. L. Hampton (Ed.), *Family violence prevention and treatment* (2nd ed.). Beverly Hills, CA: Sage.

Murphy, C., Hartman, J., Muccino, L., & Douchis, K. (1995, November). *Dependency characteristics and abusive behavior in dating relationships.* Presented at the Association for the Advancement of Behavior Therapy, Washington, DC.

Murphy, C. M., Meyer, S. L., & O'Leary, K. D. (1994). Dependency characteristics of partner assaultive men. *Journal of Abnormal Psychology, 103,* 729-735.

Murphy, C. M., & O'Leary, K. D. (1989). Psychological aggression predicts physical aggression in early marriage. *Journal of Consulting and Clinical Psychology, 57,* 579-582.

O'Leary, K. D., & Cascardi, M. (1998). Physical aggression in marriage: A developmental analysis. In T. Bradbury (Ed.), *The developmental course of marital dysfunction.* New York: Cambridge University Press.

O'Leary, K. D., & Curley, A. D. (1986). Assertion and family violence: Correlates of spouse abuse. *Journal of Marital and Family Therapy, 12,* 281-289.

O'Leary, K. D., Malone, J., & Tyree, A. (1994). Physical aggression in early marriage: Prerelationship and relationship effects. *Journal of Consulting and Clinical Psychology, 62,* 594-602.

Paulhus, D. L. (1991). *Balanced Inventory of Desirable Responding reference manual for version 6.* Vancouver: University of British Columbia.

Rathus, J. H. (1994). *Attachment, coercive control, and wife abuse.* Unpublished Doctoral Dissertation, State University of New York at Stony Brook.

Riggs, D. S., Murphy, C. M., & O'Leary, K. D. (1989). Intentional falsification in reports of interpartner aggression. *Journal of Interpersonal Violence, 4,* 220-232.

Rodenburg, F. A., & Fantuzzo, J. W. (1993). The measure of wife abuse: Steps toward the development of a comprehensive assessment technique. *Journal of Family Violence, 8,* 203-228.

Romero, M. (1985). A comparison between strategies used on prisoners of war and battered wives. *Sex Roles, 13,* 537-547.

Scott, E. S. (1995). *Wife battering in light of attachment theory.* Unpublished Master's thesis. University of Maryland, Baltimore County.

Snedecor, G. W., & Cochran, W. G. (1980). *Statistical methods* (7th ed.). Ames, Iowa: Iowa State University Press.

Straus, M. A. (1979). Measuring intrafamily conflict and violence: The Conflict Tactics Scales. *Journal of Marriage and the Family, 41,* 75-88.

Straus, M. A. (1990). The Conflict Tactics Scales and its critics: An evaluation and new data on validity and reliability. In M. A. Straus & R. J. Gelles (Eds.), *Physical violence in American families* (pp. 49-73). New Brunswick, NJ: Transaction.

Straus, M. A., Hamby, S. L., Boney-McCoy, S., & Sugarman, D. B. (1996). The revised conflict tactics scales (CTS2): Development and preliminary psychometric data. *Journal of Family Issues, 17,* 283-316.

Sugarman, D. B., & Hotaling, G. T. (1989). Dating violence: Prevalence, context, and risk markers. In M. A. Pirog-Good & J. E. Stets (Eds.), *Violence in dating relationships: Emerging social issues.* New York: Praeger.

Sugarman, D. B., & Hotaling, G. T. (1997). Intimate violence and social desirability: A meta-analytic review. *Journal of Interpersonal Violence, 12,* 275-290.

Tolman, R. M. (1989). The development of a measure of psychological maltreatment of women by their male partners. *Violence and Victims, 4,* 159-177.

West, M. L., & Sheldon-Keller, A. E. (1994). *Patterns of relating: An adult attachment perspective.* New York: Guilford.

Wiggins, J. S., Phillips, N., & Trapnell, P. (1989). Circular reasoning about interpersonal behavior: Evidence concerning some untested assumptions underlying diagnostic classification. *Journal of Personality and Social Psychology, 56,* 296-305.

Wiggins, J. S., Trapnell, P., & Phillips, N. (1988). Psychometric and geometric characteristics of the revised Interpersonal Adjective Scales (IAS-R). *Multivariate Behavioral Research, 23,* 517-530.

NOTE

[1]The original 34 items were adapted or selected from an unpublished item set provided by Everett Waters from his research on attachment in early marriage, Tolman's (1989) Psychological Maltreatment of Women Inventory which was developed for use with clinical domestic violence samples, the psychological aggression items from Straus's Conflict Tactics Scale (Straus, 1979), an item set designed to assess fear-producing and dependency-producing abusive behaviors among clinical sample batterers (Scott, 1995), and items generated by a discussion group of undergraduate research assistants.

Chapter 3

The Validation of the Psychological Maltreatment of Women Inventory

Richard M. Tolman

P sychological maltreatment has only recently begun to receive the attention of family violence researchers. The study of psychological maltreatment is important for several reasons. Evidence suggests that psychological maltreatment almost always accompanies physical abuse. A study by Stets (1990) found that 99% of battered women experienced some type of emotional abuse as measured by the verbal aggression scale of the Conflict Tactics Scale (CTS). Follingstad, Rutledge, and Hanse (1990) also found 99% of battered women in their sample experienced psychological maltreatment, and 72% experienced at least four different types of abuse. Psychological maltreatment may be an important predictor of subsequent physical violence. For example, Murphy and O'Leary (1989) reported that a husband's use of psychological aggression at 18 months after marriage significantly predicted subsequent physical aggression 1 year later. Further, the clinical literature and some preliminary research evidence suggests that psychological maltreatment itself may be as detrimental as physical abuse (Follingstad et al., 1990; Murphy & Cascardi, 1999; Tolman & Bhosley, 1991).

A number of approaches to measurement of psychological maltreatment have emerged, perhaps reflecting the growing interest in research on psychological maltreatment. The most widely used measure has been the verbal aggression scale of the CTS (Straus, 1979). The CTS has only a limited numbers of items, tapping a narrow domain of psychological maltreatment. More recently, a number of measures with broader item domains have been developed. Among the measures with subscales measuring psychological maltreatment are the Index of Spouse Abuse (Hudson & McIntosh, 1981), the Abusive Behavior Inventory (Shepard & Campbell, 1992), and the Severity of Violence Against Women Scales (Marshall, 1992). This study provides some evidence for the validity of one approach to measurement of psychological maltreatment, the Psychological Maltreatment of Women Inventory (PMWI, Tolman, 1989).

BACKGROUND ON PMWI

The PMWI is a 58-item instrument designed to measure the level of psychological maltreatment of women by their male partners in intimate relationships. Previous work (Tolman, 1989) demonstrated a high rate of endorsement of the items by battered women and men who batter. In addition, the study established a factor structure which resulted in two internally consistent subscales labeled Dominance-Isolation (e.g., my partner was jealous or suspicious of my friends; my partner restricted my use of the telephone) and Emotional-Verbal (e.g., my partner blamed me for his problems; my partner told me my feelings were irrational or crazy). Consistent with results of self-reports of physical abuse (Browning & Dutton, 1986; Edleson & Brygger, 1986; Jouriles & O'Leary, 1985; Szinovacz, 1983), men underreported psychological maltreatment when partners' reports were used as a criterion.

PURPOSE OF THIS STUDY

This study attempts to provide evidence of the validity the PMWI in several ways. Evidence for concurrent instrument validity can be provided examining the correlations of the PMWI with other measures of psychological maltreatment. High correlations of the PMWI with variables that are theoretically related (e.g., physical abuse) demonstrate convergent validity, a form of construct validity. In addition, lower correlations with variables believed to have a modest or no relationship to psychological maltreatment (e.g., demographic variables) provides evidence for the discriminant validity of the scale.

In addition we apply an adaptation of the known-groups method for establishing the validity of a scale. This study examines if scores on the PMWI discriminate between known-groups of physically abused women and those who are not abused. The known-groups method generally is considered to establish criterion validity. However, the method applied in this study is more accurately described as a form of construct validity because the designation of known-groups is based on physical abuse rather than psychological maltreatment. Given the theoretical link between physical abuse and psychological maltreatment, psychological maltreatment scores should be higher for those who have experienced physical abuse and those who have not.

The construct validity of the PMWI can be further demonstrated by establishing that psychological maltreatment differs from related constructs. Differences on the PMWI between abused women and those who are not might be due to higher levels of relationship distress rather than to psychological maltreatment per se. Therefore, if psychological maltreatment is distinct from relationship distress, PMWI scores should be higher for those in physically abusive relationships and those in distressed but not physically abusive relationships. We predicted that psychological maltreatment would be highest in the group known to be abused. Because some level of psychological maltreatment is likely to be present in most distressed relationships, we predicted the distressed but not physically abused group would score higher than a relationship satisfied group but lower than the physically abused group.

In addition to exploration of the validity of the original scale, this study examines the reliability and validity of a short version of the PMWI. I originally intended the measure for use in batterer intervention programs, to assess which types of psychological maltreatment batterers use and to evaluate whether programs succeed in changing batterers' psychologically abusive behavior. Because of its intended clinical use, I viewed comprehensiveness as a virtue. However, the length of the measure potentially limits its use in research that attempts to measure psychological maltreatment as well as other variables. Therefore, in this study, I attempted to construct and validate a shorter version of the scale for use in settings where the full measure is not practical.

METHODS

Participants

One hundred women were recruited for participation in the study from several sources including agencies providing domestic violence services, social service agencies providing counseling and other services, hospitals, parenting classes, and through public service announcements and ads advertising a study on relationships. Participants were eligible for inclusion in the study if they had been in a cohabiting relationship for at least 1 year, and had not been separated from their partner for more than 1 month in the past 6 months.

Instruments

In addition to the PMWI each participant completed several paper and pencil measures.

Conflict Tactics Scale. The Conflict Tactics Scale (CTS; Straus, 1979) has been widely used as a measure of spouse abuse and its validity and reliability has been empirically demonstrated in a number of studies. The scale has three subscales (reasoning, verbal abuse, and physical abuse). In this study, only the physical abuse subscale was used.

Index of Marital Satisfaction. The Index of Marital Satisfaction (IMS; Cheung & Hudson, 1982; Hudson, 1982) is a 25-item instrument designed to measure the degree, severity or magnitude of problems one partner has in the relationship. The IMS has high internal consistency (.96) and has excellent concurrent validity (Corcoran & Fischer, 1988). Scores of 30 or above were used to establish evidence of relationship discord.

Index of Spouse Abuse. The Index of Spouse Abuse (ISA; Hudson & McIntosh, 1981) is a 30-item self-report measure with two subscales, one measuring physical (ISAP) and the other measuring non-physical abuse (ISA-NP) of a woman by her spouse or partner. The scale asks respondents to rate how often various abusive behaviors have occurred in their relationships.

Brief Symptom Inventory. The BSI (Derogatis & Melisaratos, 1983) contains 53 symptom items rated on a 5-point scale to reflect respondents' distress from that symptom. In this study, respondents were asked to rate their distress during the past month. The BSI yields scores for nine specific problems including somatization, obsessive-compulsive problems, interpersonal sensitivity, depression, anxiety, hostility, phobic anxiety, paranoid ideation, and psychoticism. For this study, the Global Severity Index (GSI) was used. The GSI represents the average intensity of symptoms for all items. Some studies have suggested that the BSI is unidimensional, making the use of a global scale rather than specific problem indices more appropriate (Piersma, Boes, & Reaume, 1994).

Group Classification

Based on scores on the IMS and the CTS, the 100 participants were divided into three groups: Battered women (BW, $n = 39$), women in distressed relationships who were not battered (RD, $n = 22$), and nonbattered women who were satisfied with their relationships (RS, $n = 39$). Women were classified as being in distressed relationships if their IMS score was greater than 30, the clinical cutting score established for the measure (Hudson, 1982). Women were placed in the physical abuse group if they met one of the following three criteria: (1) one or more incidents of the following: hit with an object, kicked or hit with a fist, beat up, burned, choked or strangled, physically forced to have sex;

(2) more than one incident of being pushed, carried, restrained, slapped, or spanked; (3) multiple incidents of any type of physical abuse in the past year (e.g., one incident of pushing, grabbing, and shoving, and one incident of hitting with a fist).

RESULTS

Comparability of the Groups

Analysis of the demographic characteristics of the initial sample showed the BW and RD groups did not differ significantly on any characteristic. However, the BW group was more dissimilar from the RS group, with statistically significant differences in age ($t = 2.77, p = .007$), highest grade completed ($t = -3.06, p = .003$). Overall, the RS group was younger and better educated than the BW group. Because of these demographic differences, dropping some of the RS cases created a demographically balanced comparison group. This resulted in a final sample of 83 participants. The three groups did not differ significantly from one another on any of the variables. The characteristics of the three groups used in subsequent analyses are summarized in Table 1.

Construct Validity

I examined the correlations of the scales with other measures to assess the discriminant validity of the measures. If the measure has discriminant validity, it should correlate highly with other measures of psychological maltreatment. It should also correlate relatively highly with physical abuse and more moderately with measures that are related to but distinct from psychological maltreatment, such as physical abuse, relationship distress, and psychological symptoms. Correlations with measures not believed to be strongly associated with psychological maltreatment, such as demographic variables, should be low.

Table 2 shows the correlations with various measures. As predicted, all subscales correlated highly with the nonphysical abuse subscale of the Index of Spouse Abuse. Correlations with the CTS physical abuse measure and the ISA physical abuse measure were also high, though somewhat lower than correlations with the ISA nonphysical abuse scale. Correlations with marital satisfaction were moderate to high. Correlations with the GSI were moderate. Demographic variables were not significantly related to levels of psychological maltreatment.

Group Comparisons

ANOVA analysis tested the ability of the PMWI subscales to discriminate among the three groups. I expected the BW to score significantly higher than the other two

TABLE 1. Demographic Characteristics of Sample

Group	African American	Hispanic	White	Other
Battered	10.3	5.1	82.1	2.6
Distressed/Non-Battered	31.8	4.5	63.6	0.0
Nondistressed/Non-Battered	27.7	0.0	68.2	4.5
Total	20.5	3.6	73.5	2.4

	Married		Working Full-time	
Battered	66.7		67.9	
Distressed	77.3		81.0	
Nondistressed	68.2		73.3	
Total	69.0		73.4	

Group	Age	# of Children	Months Known Partner	Highest Grade
Battered ($n = 38$)	37.0	1.8	109.6	13.8
Distressed ($n = 22$)	38.7	1.9	136.5	14.3
Nondistressed ($n = 22$)	34.4	1.4	128.3	14.3
Total	36.8	1.5	121.8	14.0

groups and the RD group to score higher than the RS group. Bonnferoni-Dunn contrasts revealed the BW group was higher than the RD group and the RS group, and the RD group was higher than the RS group. See Table 3.

Construction of a Short Version of the Scale

Given the evidence for the validity of the larger subscales, we used those subscale items as the basis for a construction of a short version of the PMWI. First, I tested the mean PMWI item scores for BW and RD groups. This step was an exploratory device to narrow items for selection, so we did not control for multiple comparisons. Table 4 lists the items with significant differences between the BW and RD groups. These items are likely to be the aspects of psychological maltreatment most distinct from general relationship distress.

Two seven-item scales were constructed from these items, drawn from the larger list of items, see Appendix 2. The items were chosen purposely to increase content validity for the short scale versions. The two short subscales each had excellent reliability (D/I, alpha = .88; V/E, alpha = .92).

A factor analysis using only the 14 items chosen demonstrated that the short-scale factor structure is consistent with prior work on the factor structure of the larger PMWI (Tolman, 1989). The factor loadings for the short-scale items are compared with the loadings from the previous study in Table 5.

TABLE 2. Correlations of PMWI Scales with Other Variables

Scale Version	Index of Spouse Abuse Non-Physical	Index of Spouse Abuse Physical	Conflict Tactics Scale	Index of Marital Satisfaction	Brief Symptom Inventory General Symptom Index	Years of Education	Age	Number of Children	Family Income
Dominance-Isolation Long Form	.94**	.85**	.68**	.70**	.48**	-.20	-.31*	.24	-.18
Dominance-Isolation Short Form	.88**	.86**	.68**	.62**	.46**	-.28	.27	.23	-.21
Emotional Verbal Long Form	.89**	.78**	.64**	.82**	.54***	-.22	.33*	.22	-.20
Emotional Verbal Short Form	.90**	.80**	.65**	.76**	.51**	-.24	.29*	.19	-.18

$*p < .05, **p < .01, ***p < .001.$

TABLE 3. Mean Differences Among Battered, Relationship Distressed, and Relationship Satisfied Women on PMWI Subscales

		Emotional/ Verbal		Dominance/ Isolation	
Group	n	M	SD	M	SD
Battered women (BW)	39	70.7	21.5	61.7	25.5
Relationship Distressed (RD)	22	57.0	20.0	45.4	11.8
Relationship Satisfied (RS)	22	31.9	6.2	39.3	3.2
Contrasts		I-J	S.E.	I-J	S.E.
BW(I) - RD(J)		13.7*	4.88	16.2**	4.93
BW(I) - RS(J)		38.8***	4.88	32.4***	4.93
RD(I) - RS(J)		25.1***	5.52	16.1*	5.57

$*p < .15, **p < .01, ***p < .001.$

TABLE 4. Items With Significant Differences Between Battered and Relationship Distressed Groups

10. My partner called me names.
11. My partner swore at me.
12. My partner yelled and screamed at me.
13. My partner treated me like an inferior.
26. My partner monitored my time and made me account for my hereabouts.
30. My partner used our money or made important financial decisions without talking to me about it.
32. My partner was jealous or suspicious of my friends.
35. My partner did not want me to socialize with my female friends.
36. My partner accused me of having an affair with another man.
38. My partner tried to keep me from seeing or talking to my family.
39. My partner interfered in my relationships with other family members.
40. My partner tried to keep me from doing things to help myself.
42. My partner restricted my use of the telephone.
43. My partner did not allow me to leave the house.
44. My partner did not allow me to work.
45. My partner told me my feelings were irrational or crazy.
46. My partner blamed me for his problems.
47. My partner tried to turn my family against me.
49. My partner tried to make me feel crazy.
50. My partner's moods changed radically.
51. My partner blamed me when he was upset, even if I had nothing to do with it.
53. My partner threatened to hurt himself if I left.
58. My partner threatened to commit me to an institution.

$p < .05.$

Given the reliability and factorial validity of the short subscales, the subscales were analyzed to determine their ability to differentiate between the groups. Using ANOVA, with Bonnferoni-Dunn contrasts, the BW group scored significantly higher than the RD, the BW group scored higher than the RS group, and the RD scored higher than the RS group. See Table 6.

TABLE 5. Factor Structure of Short Version

| | Loading in Study 2 | | Item Loading in Study of Entire Measure | | | |
	Emot	Dom	Emot	Rank (of 24)	Dom	Rank (of 26)
PMWI 12	.80	.30	.60	11		
PMWI 13	.78	.39	.63	7		
PMWI 45	.78	.14	.63	8		
PMWI 49	.77	.42	.61	10		
PMWI 11	.75	.37	.54	16		
PMWI 46	.67	.53	.71	1		
PMWI 10	.65	.56	.47	20		
PMWI 36	.19	.82			.59	15
PMWI 39	.25	.79			.70	5
PMWI 26	.30	.76			.75	1
PMWI 40	.36	.71			.75	2
PMWI 30	.40	.61			.48	22
PMWI 32	.49	.59			.67	9
PMWI 42	.41	.53			.67	8

TABLE 6. Mean Differences Among Battered, Relationship Distressed, and Relationship Satisfied Women on Short Subscales

| | | Short Emotional/ Verbal | | Short Dominance/ Isolation | |
| | | | | | |
Group	n	M	SD	M	SD
Battered women (BW)	39	21.2	7.7	17.2	7.5
Relationship Distressed (RD)	22	15.0	6.0	11.0	3.7
Relationship Satisfied (RS)	22	8.7	2.1	8.0	1.4
Contrasts		I-J	S.E.	I-J	S.E.
BW(I) - RD(J)		6.2*	1.66	6.3***	1.49
BW(I) - RS(J)		12.5***	1.66	9.2***	1.49
RD(I) - RS(J)		6.3**	1.88	2.9	1.68

*p < .=05, **p < .01, ***p < .001.

Differentiating Between Service-Seeking and Community Sample of Battered Women

To test the construct validity of the long and short scales, I divided the battered women into two groups, those recruited from the community and those recruited from agencies providing service to battered women. This resulted in four demographically balanced comparison groups, service-seeking battered women (SB), battered women recruited from the community (CB), maritally distressed nonbattered women (RD), and the nonbattered, nondistressed community sample (RS).

I utilized ANOVA analysis to determine the ability of both the long and short versions of the emotional/verbal and dominance isolation scales to differentiate among the four groups. Pairwise contrasts (Bonferroni-Dunn) revealed that the SB group differed significantly form the RD and RS groups for all four scales. The CB group differed significantly from the RS group on all four measures. However, the CB group did not differ from the RD group on any measures.

DISCUSSION

This study provides some evidence for the validity of the PMWI and the shorter subscales derived from it. All PMWI subscales correlate highly with the physical abuse scale of the ISA and the physical abuse subscale from the CTS. The discriminant validity of the subscales is supported by the pattern of correlations with other measures. The results provide evidence for construct validity because battered women scored significantly higher than women in distressed but nonbattering relationships on both subscales. This assumes that battered women are more likely to be psychologically abused than women in distressed nonbattering relationships.

The evidence for validity is clouded, however, by the analysis of the separate shelter and community subgroups of battered women. Service-seeking battered women differ significantly from both nonservice seeking battered women and nonbattered women in distressed relationships. There was no significant difference on either PMWI subscale between nonservice seeking battered and nonbattered women in distressed relationships (see Table 7). There are three possible explanations. One explanation is that the PMWI does not measure a construct distinct from relationship distress. A second explanation is that women in distressed relationships experience as much psychological maltreatment as those in physically abusive relationships. There is evidence to suggest that psychological maltreatment is common in distressed marriages. For example, Barling, O'Leary, Jouriles, Vivian, and MacEwen (1987), report that at least 89% of couples entering marital therapy report some of the verbal aggression items from the CTS. A third explanation calls into question the validity of the group categories. Assigning women to battered and nonbattered groups based on reports in the past year of multiple incidents of physical abuse or severe abuse may have been an inadequate method for distinguishing

TABLE 7. Mean Differences Among Service-Seeking Battered, Nonservice-Seeking Battered, Relationship Distressed, and Relationship Satisfied Women on PMWI Subscales

Group	n	Short Emotional/ Verbal		Short Dominance/ Isolation		Dominance/ Isolation		Emotional/ Verbal	
		M	SD	M	SD	M	SD	M	SD
Service-Seeking Battered (SS)	18	25.6	5.7	20.3	6.4	72.3	23.0	84.9	13.0
Nonservice Seeking Battered (CB)	21	17.4	7.2	14.6	7.45	52.6	24.0	58.5	20.0
Relationship Distressed (RD)	22	15.0	60.0	11.0	3.7	45.4	11.8	57.0	20.0
Relationship Satisfied (RS)	22	8.7	2.1	8.0	1.4	29.3	3.2	31.9	6.2
Contrasts		I-J	S.E.	I-J	S.E.	I-J	S.E.	I-J	S.E.
SS(I) - CB(J)		8.1***	1.79	5.8**	1.68	19.7*	5.55	26.4***	40.27
SS(I) - RD(J)		10.6***	1.77	9.4***	1.66	26.9**	5.49	28.0***	41.60
SS(I) - RS(J)		16.9***	1.77	12.3***	1.66	43.0***	5.49	53.0***	66.74
CB(I) - RD(J)		2.4	1.70	.36	1.60	7.21	5.27	1.5	4.86
CB(I) - RS(J)		8.7***	1.70	6.5**	1.60	23.3***	5.27	26.6***	4.80
RD(I) - RS(J)		6.3*	1.68	2.9	1.58	16.1*	5.21	25.1***	4.80

$*p < .05, **p < .01, ***p < .001.$

between those groups. Some women in the RD group had experienced single acts of less severe physical abuse in the past year, and some may have been abused in the past. As a result, the CB group may be more similar to the RD group than we intended.

A comparison of known groups of psychologically maltreated nonbattered women with women who have not been psychologically maltreated would provide stronger evidence of criterion validity. Unfortunately, it is difficult to recruit a sample of women who are known to experience only psychological maltreatment. Currently, there is no "gold standard" for determining whether someone is experiencing psychological maltreatment other than their subjective global report. My experience, and that of others (Loring, 1994), has been that even some women who report frequent and pervasive acts of maltreatment do not necessarily label themselves as psychologically maltreated, further complicating studies attempting to validate a measure of psychological maltreatment based on a known-groups method.

An additional caution must be raised about the construct validity of the short subscales. Because they are derived from items that differed significantly between the BW and RD groups, the significant subscale differences may be inflated by type 1 error. A cross validation study is necessary to see if these differences are replicated on other samples to enhance confidence in the validity of the short-version subscales. While the short-version subscales may prove to be useful for establishing levels of psychological maltreatment in research, caution should be exercised in their clinical use. Because of their length, they do not adequately sample from all relevant domains of maltreatment. They might prove useful as a quick screening device, which could be followed up with more extensive clinical interviewing.

It is premature to set any PMWI cutting score as establishing clinical evidence for the existence of psychological maltreatment. This validation sample is small, and further research with more representative populations is necessary to determine what levels of psychological maltreatment clearly distinguish between abusive and nonabusive relationships.

REFERENCES

Barling, J., O'Leary, K. D., Jouriles, E. N., Vivian, D., & MacEwen, K. E. (1987). Factor similarity of the Conflict Tactics Scales across samples, spouses, and sites: Issues and implications. *Journal of Family Violence, 2,* 37-54.

Browning, J., & Dutton, D. (1986). Assessment of wife assault with the Conflict Tactics Scale: Using couple data to quantify the differential reporting effect. *Journal of Marriage and the Family, 48*(2), 375-379.

Cheung, P. P., & Hudson, W. W. (1982). Assessment of marital discord in social work practice: A revalidation of the Index of Marital Satisfaction. *Journal of Social Service Research, 5*(1-2), 101-118.

Corcoran, K., & Fischer, J. (1987). *Measures for Clinical Practice.* New York: The Free Press.

Derogatis, L. R., & Melisaratos, N. (1983). The Brief Symptom Inventory: An introductory report. *Psychological Medicine, 13*(3), 599-605.

Edleson, J. L., & Brygger, M. (1986). Gender differences in reporting of battering incidents. *Family Relations, 35,* 377-382.

Follingstad, D. R., Rutledge, L. L., Berg, B. J., & Hause, E. S. (1990). The role of emotional abuse in physically abusive relationships. *Journal of Family Violence, 5*(2), 107-120.

Hudson, W. W. (1982). A measurement package for clinical workers. *Journal of Applied Behavioral Science, 18*(2), 229-238.

Hudson, W. W., & McIntosh, S. R. (1981). The assessment of spouse abuse: Two quantifiable dimensions. *Journal of Marriage and the Family, 43,* 873-885.

Jouriles, E. N., & O'Leary, K. D. (1985). Interspousal reliability of reports of marital violence. *Journal of Consulting & Clinical Psychology, 53*(3), 419-421.

Loring, M. (1994). *Emotional abuse.* New York: Lexington Books.

Marshall, L. L. (1992). Development of the Severity of Violence Against Women Scales. *Journal of Family Violence, 7*(2), 103-121.

Murphy, C. M., & Cascardi, M. (1999). Psychological aggression and abuse in marriage. In R. L. Hampton (Ed.), *Issues in Children's and Families' Lives* (2nd ed.). Beverly Hills: Sage.

Murphy, C. M., & O'Leary, K. D. (1989). Psychological aggression predicts physical aggression in early marriage. *Journal of Consulting and Clinical Psychology, 57*(5), 579-582.

Piersma, H., Boes, J., & Reaume, W. (1994). Unidimensionality of the Brief Symptom Inventory (BSI) in adult and adolescent inpatients. *Journal of Personality Assessment, 63*(2), 338-344

Shepard, M., & Campbell, J. (1992). The abusive behavior inventory: A measure of psychological and physical abuse. *Journal of Interpersonal Violence, 7*(3), 291-305.

Stets, J. (1990). Verbal and physical aggression in marriage. *Journal of Marriage and the Family, 52*(2), 501-514.

Straus, M. A. (1979). Measuring intrafamilial conflict and violence: The conflict tactics (CT) scale. *Journal of Marriage and the Family, 45,* 75-78.

Szinovacz, M. (1983). Using couple data as a methodological tool: The case of marital violence. *Journal of Marriage and the Family, 45,* 633-644.

Tolman, R. M. (1989). The development of a measure of psychological maltreatment of women by their male partners. *Violence and Victims, 4*(3), 173-189.

Tolman, R. M., & Bhosley, G. (1991). The outcome of participation in shelter-sponsored program for men who batter. In D. Knudsen & J. Miller (Eds.), *Abused and battered: Social and legal responses to family violence* (pp. 113-122). Hawthorne, NY: Aldine de Gruyter.

Chapter 4

The Dominance Scale:
Preliminary Psychometric
Properties

Sherry L. Hamby

M ale dominance may be the most widely mentioned risk factor for physical
assaults on an intimate partner (e.g., Campbell, 1992; Coleman & Straus,
1986; Frieze & McHugh, 1992; Gelles, 1983; Koss et al., 1994; Stets,
1992; Yllö, 1984). Dominance is perhaps most closely associated with feminism
and feminist theories of domestic violence (e.g., Dobash & Dobash, 1979; Yllö &
Bograd, 1988), but it is also a primary construct in numerous other theoretical
models of partner violence. These include resource theory (Allen & Straus, 1980;
Goode, 1971), exchange/social control theory (Gelles, 1983), status incompatibility
theory (Hornung, McCullough, & Sugimoto, 1981), and some psychological
models (e.g., Dutton & Strachan, 1987; Haj-Yahia & Edleson, 1994). Dominance
plays very different roles across these theories, however. In fact, in some theories,
greater dominance is hypothesized to cause more violence (e.g., Gelles, 1983; Yllö
& Bograd, 1988), while in others, it is lack of power that is hypothesized to cause
violence (e.g., Dutton, 1994; Goode, 1971).

A new conceptualization of dominance has been offered (Hamby, 1996) that
further explicates the links between dominance and partner violence. This
chapter establishes preliminary psychometric properties for a scale that is
consistent with this reformulation. Three different forms of dominance are

outlined in this new conceptualization: authority, restrictiveness, and dispar-agement. Each can perhaps best be defined as one kind of deviation from an egalitarian relationship. Authority is closely related to decision-making power. In this pattern, instead of both partners in a relationship having equal input on decisions about the relationship, one partner holds a majority of decision-making power. He or she is 'in charge' of the relationship. This form of dominance is most congruent with an existing set of social norms, that of the traditional husband-led couple, but also most incongruent with another norm, that of the modern egalitarian couple. Restrictiveness departs from an egalitar-ian concept of equal individuals. One partner feels the right to intrude upon the other's behavior, even when that behavior does not directly involve the restrictive partner, as when restrictive partners prohibit their partners from spending time with certain individuals or going certain places. Disparagement occurs when one partner fails to equally value the other partner and has an overall negative appraisal of his or her partner's worth.

In this formulation, the three forms of dominance are seen as causes of partner violence (including physical and psychological aggression), not as violence in and of itself, following the majority of studies on dominance and partner violence. Many adverse outcomes result from hierarchical partner relationships, including, in addition to partner aggression, relationship dis-cord, child maltreatment, low self-esteem, depression, and others. Traditional husband-led couples provide an example of relationships that are characterized by dominance but are not universally aggressive. Both dominance and aggres-sion are typical of batterers (e.g., Johnson, 1995), and both are associated with distress when found in adult intimate relationships (for reviews of each construct, see Gray-Little & Burks, 1983; Koss et al., 1994).

In the partner violence literature, most existing measures of dominance assess either Authority or Restrictiveness. For example, the various versions that exist of the Blood and Wolfe scale (1960), which asks about decision-making power, can be considered measures of Authority, as can some alternatives, such as the scale used by Spitzberg and Marshall (1991). Data on the association of such measures with partner violence has produced mixed results (Hotaling & Sugarman, 1986). Restrictiveness has been assessed most commonly in studies of courtship violence, using instruments such as the Interpersonal Control scale (Stets & Pirog-Good, 1990) and the Dominance-Possessiveness index (Rouse, 1990). In these studies, a positive association was found between dominance and partner violence, suggest-ing that this kind of dominance may be more intimately linked with violent behavior. This may be because of the intolerance that is especially characteristic of restrictive partners.

The third form of dominance, disparagement, has received less attention in the dominance literature, even though these kinds of hypercritical downward social comparisons are an important way in which individuals elevate them-selves with respect to their partners (cf. Wills, 1981). Disparagement should not be confused with more commonly studied attitudes toward women (e.g., Haj-Yahia & Edleson, 1994), in that it refers specifically to attitudes toward one's own partner and is not necessarily gender-specific. This idea has been included in some measures of dominance, such as the Dominance Motive index ('I want my partner to know that I am stronger or better at some things than he/she is,') (Rouse, 1990).

In this study, a new scale to assess each of these different forms of dominance was evaluated. One important advantage to this new scale is the ability to compare the associations of different dominance patterns with constructs of interest, such as partner violence. Preliminary psychometric data on the three subscales using an undergraduate sample are presented and these scores are compared to other variables of interest. It was predicted that Authority would be most closely related to a traditional Blood and Wolfe-style measure of dominance. Second, it was hypothesized that Restrictiveness and Disparagement would be more closely related to two response biases, social desirability and willingness to self-disclose, than Authority, because Authority deviates less from some (traditional) societal norms. Finally, the associations of these different subscales to partner violence were examined and it was hypothesized that Restrictiveness would be more closely associated with partner violence than Authority, following the patterns observed in other studies.

METHOD

Participants

The participants were 131 male and female undergraduates attending one of two colleges in the Northeast, one of which is oriented toward older, nontraditional students. Participants were volunteers who were recruited through undergraduate sociology and justice studies courses. Most students were White and came from intact families with upper middle socioeconomic status. Most participants provided information about dating (noncohabiting) relationships, although almost a quarter of the sample reported that they lived with their partner. The demographics of the sample are outlined in more detail in Table 1.

Measures

Participants first provided the demographic information referred to above and in Table 1.

The Dominance Scale. Thirty-seven items were tested for the Dominance Scale. Items were generated by a team of people with research and clinical experience who were familiar with other scales in the field and were reviewed for awkward wording by a different sample of 97 undergraduates. Items that could be answered yes or no

**TABLE 1. Respondents' Sociodemographic and
Relationship Characteristics**

Sex		Relationship status	
Female	61%	Dating	82%
Male	39%	Engaged	4%
Age (in years)		Married	14%
Mean	24.00	Cohabiting	
(*SD*)	(7.62)	No	76%
Ethnic Identity		Yes	24%
Caucasian	99%	Relationship length	
Hispanic	1%	1 to 5 months	25%
Family's personal income		6 to 12 months	16%
(yearly estimated)		> 1 to 2 years	22%
Under $39,999	19%	More than 2 years	37%
$40,000-$59,999	26%	Current or past relationship	
$60,000-$79,999	26%	Current	70%
Over $80,000	29%	Past (ended within last year)	30%

were avoided. The item pool covered three theoretical areas: 14 items assessed Authority, 12 assessed Restrictiveness, and 11 assessed Disparagement. Respondents were asked to indicate how much they agreed or disagreed (on a 4-point scale) with each item. Each subscale was scored so that higher scores reflected more dominant behavior; some items were reverse scored. (See results of factor analyses for more information. The final scale has a Flesch reading level of grade 7.4. See Appendix for the final version of the scale.)

Decision-Making in Intimate Relationships Scale (DMIR; Hamby, 1992). The DMIR is an 11-item scale in the format first used by Blood and Wolfe (1960), but modified so that it is appropriate for use with cohabiting and noncohabiting couples. For each of 11 specific contents areas (e.g., what to do on weekends, when to have sex), participants indicate who usually has the final say in that area on a 5-point scale (partner always, partner usually, equal, you usually, you always). Higher scores indicate more decision-making power resides with the participant.

Jourard Self-Disclosure Questionnaire (JSDQ; Jourard, 1971; Raphael & Dohrenwend, 1987). A 27-item version of the Jourard Self-Disclosure Questionnaire was used that Raphael & Dohrenwend developed to avoid confounding disclosure with psychopathology. Participants indicated on a 4-point scale how much they have disclosed to casual friends about various topics. "Casual friends" was chosen as the target individual (numerous targets have been used in the past) to assess how likely participants would disclose personal information to nonintimate individuals, as they are asked to do on questionnaires. Higher scores indicate greater self-disclosure.

Conflict Tactics Scale, Revised (CTS2; Straus, Hamby, Boney-McCoy, & Sugarman, 1996). An extended 120-item version of the CTS2 was administered.

Scores were obtained for Negotiation (positive conflict resolution tactics), Psychological Aggression, Physical Assault, and Injury. Participants were asked to report on both their own and their partner's violent behavior during the past year, resulting in eight separate subscale scores. Almost all participants (91%) reported using psychological aggression, 38% reported they had physically assaulted their partner, and 14% that they had caused pain or injury. Their reports of sustaining aggression were similar: 90% reported sustaining psychological aggression, 36% reported sustaining physical assault, and 18% reported sustaining injury. The overlap between inflicted and sustained aggression was high; 88% reported both for psychological aggression, 31% reported both for physical assault, and 11% reported both for injury.

Marlowe-Crowne Social Desirability Scale (MCSD; Crowne & Marlowe, 1960). This is a 33-item true-false test that measures an unwillingness to acknowledge negative traits. Higher scores indicate greater tendencies to respond in socially desirable ways.

Procedure

Data were collected during the regular class period of eight undergraduate classes. Students were informed of the purpose of the study and that their decision to participate or not would have no influence on their class grade. All questionnaires were completed during class time. No one returned a blank questionnaire, resulting in a total collection of 164 questionnaires. Participants who had never been in a relationship were asked to describe their parents' relationship where applicable; these students (1%) were dropped from all analyses. Participants who indicated they had ended their last relationship more than one year ago (9%) were also dropped, as were any individuals who omitted any question on the Dominance Scale (10%), resulting in a final sample of 131. Omissions on the Dominance Scale did not show any clear pattern and dropped participants did not differ in aggressiveness from retained ones, $p > .10$. Participants were debriefed further after completing the questionnaire and provided a list of shelters, clinics, and other locally available mental health services.

RESULTS

Factor Analysis of Subscales

The sample size is not sufficient to factor analyze the entire Dominance Scale item pool, so separate factor analyses were conducted for each theoretical subscale, Authority, Restrictiveness, and Disparagement. Each analysis was a principal factors analysis using squared multiple correlations to estimate communalities (this approach assumes the presence of error in the data, unlike a principal components analysis). These analyses provide information on the internal construct validity of each subscale, and can identify items that are not similar to others on these subscales, but they do not provide information on the overlap among subscales.

Authority. The first factor accounted for a very high percentage of the variance in these 14 items (83%), so a one-factor solution was retained for these data. Two items, "I know what's best for my partner," and "I expect my partner to listen to what I say without arguing," did not load at the .3 level and were dropped. The other 12 items, however, had generally high loadings and were retained; the alpha for these items was .80. The distribution of this scale was approximately normal, although more scores clustered closer to the mean than would be expected. See Table 2 for the items, factor loadings, and final communality estimates for this subscale.

Restrictiveness. A one-factor solution again accounted for most of the variance (82%) in these 12 items. All but three items, "I respect my partner's need for privacy," "I can meet all of my partner's emotional needs," and "I am controlling in my relationship with my partner," loaded on this factor, resulting in a 9-item subscale with a coefficient alpha of .73. The distribution of this scale was approximately normal. The items, factor loadings, and final communality estimates for this subscale are also in Table 2.

Disparagement. The first factor accounted for 87% of the variance of these 11 items, which are listed in Table 2. Thus, a one-factor solution was accepted. All 11 items had loadings that were at least .30, so no item was deleted from this subscale. The resulting subscale had a coefficient alpha of .82. The distribution of this scale was approximately normal. The individual loadings and final communality estimates can also be found in Table 2.

Intercorrelations Among Subscales

The highest intercorrelation occurred between Authority and Disparagement. Authority and Restrictiveness were moderately correlated, and Disparagement and Restrictiveness were not correlated. The patterns of correlations for males and females were not significantly different from each other and were therefore combined. See Table 3 for the correlations for the entire sample. The means and standard deviations for the subscales are also in this table.

Associations With Other Constructs

Correlations of the three subscales with the DMIR, JSDQ, and MCSD scales are in Table 4. The results of t-tests comparing the magnitude of the correlations (Bruning & Kintz, 1987) indicated that the subscales are differentially related to these constructs. As predicted, the DMIR was more highly correlated with Authority than Restrictiveness [t (128) = 5.40, $p < .01$]. Contrary to prediction, however, it was not more related to Authority than to Disparagement [t (128) = 1.62, $p > .05$], although the difference is in the hypothesized direction. Self-disclosure, as measured by the

TABLE 2. Items, Factor Loadings, and Communality Estimates for Dominance Subscales

Item	Factor Loading	Communality Estimate
Authority (alpha = .80)		
15) Sometimes I have to remind my partner of who's boss.	.71	.50
10) My partner and I generally have equal say about decisions. (R)	.67	.44
21) My partner needs to remember that I am in charge.	.65	.42
19) If my partner and I can't agree, I should have the final say.	.63	.40
31) I dominate my partner.	.56	.31
14) Things are easier in my relationship if I am in charge.	.48	.23
18) Both partners in a relationship should have equal say about decisions. (R)	.47	.22
30) I often tell my partner how to do something.	.47	.22
6) I hate losing arguments with my partner.	.46	.21
3) If my partner and I can't agree, I usually have the final say.	.44	.19
11) It would bother me if my partner made more money than I did.	.36	.13
9) When my partner and I watch TV, I hold the remote control.	.31	.09
—) I know what's best for my partner.	.29	.09
—) I expect my partner to listen to what I say without arguing.	.26	.07
Restrictiveness (alpha = .73)		
16) I have a right to know everything my partner does.	.68	.45
8) I insist on knowing where my partner is at all times.	.64	.41
32) I have a right to be involved with anything my partner does.	.54	.29
2) I try to keep my partner from spending time with opposite sex friends.	.53	.28
17) It would make me mad if my partner did something I had said not to do.	.50	.25
13) I tend to be jealous.	.47	.22
7) My partner should not keep any secrets from me.	.42	.17
20) I understand there are some things my partner may not want to talk about with me. (R)	.33	.11
4) It bothers me when my partner makes plans without talking to me first.	.30	.09
—) I am controlling in my relationship with my partner.	.26	.07
—) I can meet all my partner's emotional needs.	.19	.04
—) I respect my partner's need for privacy. (R)	.12	.01
Disparagement (alpha = .82)		
28) My partner is basically a good person. (R)	.72	.52
24) People usually like my partner. (R)	.67	.45
5) My partner doesn't have enough sense to make important decisions.	.65	.42
22) My partner is a talented person. (R)	.65	.42
1) My partner often has good ideas. (R)	.60	.37
29) My partner doesn't know how to act in public.	.56	.31
26) My partner can handle most things that happen. (R)	.55	.31
27) I sometimes think my partner is unattractive.	.55	.31
25) My partner makes a lot of mistakes.	.48	.23
23) It's hard for my partner to learn new things.	.40	.16
12) I generally consider my partner's interests as much as mine. (R)	.35	.12

Note. (R) indicates item should be reverse-scored.
Items have been renumbered to match reduced scale (based on factor analyses).

TABLE 3. Intercorrelations Among Subscales

	Authority	Restrictiveness	Disparagement
Authority	1.00	.38[****]	.58[****]
Restrictiveness		1.00	.03
Disparagement			1.00
Mean	22.82	20.92	17.50
Standard deviations	4.61	3.80	4.31

[****]$p < .0001$.

**TABLE 4. Correlation of Dominance Subscales
With DMIR, MCSD, JSDQ, and CTS2 Scales**

	Authority	Restrictiveness	Disparagement
DMIR	.39[****]	-.08	.27[**]
MCSD	-.35[****]	-.14	-.18[*]
ISDQ	.02	.26[**]	-.08
CTS2—Own Behavior			
Negotiation	-.22[*]	.09	-.21[*]
Psychological Aggression	.35[****]	.33[****]	.22[*]
Physical Assault	.16	.33[****]	.10
Injury	.11	.21[*]	.02
CTS2—Partner's Behavior			
Negotiation	-.19[*]	.11	-.25[**]
Psychological Aggression	.23[**]	.24[**]	.19[**]
Physical Assault	.18[*]	.22[**]	.18[*]
Injury	.11	.21[*]	.07

Note. DMIR = Decision Making in Intimate Relationships scale; MCSD = Marlowe-Crowne Social Disability scale; JSDQ = Journard Self-Disclosure Questionnaire; CTS2 = Revised Conflict Tactics Scales.
$N = 131$. [*]$p < .05$. [**]$p < .01$. [***]$p < .001$. [****]$p < .0001$.

JSDQ, was more highly correlated with Restrictiveness than with either Disparagement or Authority [$t (128) = 2.89, p < .01$, and $t (128) = 2.55, p < .05$, respectively], as predicted. Social desirability was more highly correlated with Authority than with Disparagement [$t (127) = 2.25, p < .05$] or Restrictiveness [$t (127) = 2.29, p < .05$], contrary to prediction.

Bivariate Correlations With CTS2 Scales

The correlations of each dominance subscale with each CTS2 scale are also in Table 6. All of the dominance scales were correlated in the predicted directions with measures of aggression and violence, although the magnitude differed.

Regression Models of CTS2 Scales

To identify the best set of predictors for different kinds of partner aggression, the three Dominance Scale subscales, plus the JSDQ and MCSD, were used as predictor variables in a series of regressions that treated each CTS2 scale (Negotiation, Psychological Abuse, Physical Assault, and Injury) as a dependent variable. The regressions were done on participants' reports of their own and their partner's behaviors. Thus, the latter set of equations tests how much their own dominance is associated with receiving negotiation and aggression. The JSDQ and MCSD were included as predictors because some dominance subscales had significant correlations with these measures of response bias. These simultaneous regressions measure the unique contribution of each variable after all other variables have been considered. Sex differences in the slopes of the Dominance subscales were examined, but none were found ($p > .05$ for all eight CTS2 scales), so the entire sample was used in each regression.

Only Authority was significantly associated with participants' own Negotiation scores in the regression equations; less Authority was associated with more use of Negotiation. Restrictiveness was associated with more aggression than any other variable; it was positively associated with participants' inflicted psychological aggression, physical assault, and injury. Participants' higher Restrictiveness scores were also associated with their report of greater sustained psychological aggression, physical assault ($p = .053$), and injury at the hands of their partner. Higher disparagement was only associated with greater sustained physical assault.

The measures of response bias were also associated with some CTS2 variables. A greater willingness to self-disclose (JSDQ) was associated with more Negotiation (both self and partners' behavior). Higher social desirability (MCSD) scores were associated with lower reports of psychological aggression for both self and partner reports. See Tables 5 and 6 for the results of the regression analyses.

DISCUSSION

Conclusions

Preliminary psychometric data provided support for the internal consistency of each of the dominance constructs: Authority, Restrictiveness, and Disparagement. The data also suggest that there may be important differences among dominance patterns. Further analyses indicated that Authority is most closely related to a traditional measure of decision-making power, although Disparagement was also related to decision-making power. Willingness to self-disclose was related, as hypothesized, to Restrictiveness scores, but was not associated with the other two constructs. Surprisingly, a socially desirable response bias was more closely related to Authority than to either Restrictiveness or Disparagement, although the latter

TABLE 5. Dominance, Social Desirability, and Self-Disclosure as Predictors of CTS2 Subscales—Respondents' Behavior

Variable	B	SE	β	R^2
Negotiation				
Authority	-.79	.33	-.29*	.13
Restrictiveness	.37	.30	.12	
Disparagement	0.01	0.30	.00	
Self-Disclosure (JSDQ)	4.75	1.86	.23*	
Social Desirability (SD)	-0.13	0.21	-.06	
Psychological Abuse				
Authority	0.16	0.27	.07	.21
Restrictiveness	0.70	0.24	.26**	
Disparagement	0.26	0.25	.11	
Self-Disclosure (JSDQ)	-0.62	1.52	-.03	
Social Desirability (SD)	-0.50	0.17	-.26**	
Physical Assault				
Authority	-0.08	0.13	-.07	.14
Restrictiveness	0.43	0.12	.35***	
Disparagement	0.14	0.12	.12	
Self-Disclosure (JSDQ)	-0.56	0.75	-.06	
Social Desirability (SD)	-0.13	0.08	-.15	
Injury				
Authority	0.00	0.02	.02	.08
Restrictiveness	0.05	0.02	.21*	
Disparagement	0.03	0.02	.13	
Self-Disclosure (JSDQ)	-0.02	0.13	-.01	
Social Desirability (SD)	-0.01	0.01	-.08	

Note. For each dependent variable, the same set of predictors was used. R^2 are for full models. $^*p < .05$. $^{**}p < .01$. $^{***}p < .001$.

would seem to involve greater endorsement of negative behaviors and attitudes. On the other hand, Authority may be the form of dominance that has been most directly challenged by recent social movements and thus these relatively young participants may be most concerned about being portrayed as traditional.

The intercorrelations among the forms of dominance also support the premise that there are differences among them. The three forms were not highly intercorrelated with each other with the exception of Authority and Disparagement. Of particular note is the near-zero correlation between Restrictiveness and Disparagement. This may be due to the fact that the correspondence of Restrictiveness with societal norms is complex (Hamby, 1996). Restrictiveness is similar in some ways to the enmeshment that is often idealized in portrayals of infatuation and passionate love. Erich Fromm (1956) called this "orgiastic union" and believed it to be common and valued in Western society. On the other hand, it does go against Western ideals of

TABLE 6. Dominance, Social Desirability, and Self-Disclosure as Predictors of CTS2 Subscales—Partners' Behavior

Variable	B	SE	β	R^2
Negotiation				
Authority	-0.58	0.34	-.20	.11
Restrictiveness	0.37	0.31	.12	
Disparagement	-0.29	0.31	-.10	
Self-Disclosure (JSDQ)	3.90	1.94	.18*	
Social Desirability (SD)	-0.14	0.21	-.06	
Psychological Abuse				
Authority	-0.15	0.30	-.05	.14
Restrictiveness	0.58	0.27	.20*	
Disparagement	0.50	0.28	.19	
Self-Disclosure (JSDQ)	0.79	1.70	.04	
Social Desirability (SD)	-0.49	0.19	-.24**	
Physical Assault				
Authority	-0.12	0.15	-.10	.09
Restrictiveness	0.26	0.13	.19 ($p = .053$)	
Disparagement	0.28	0.14	.23*	
Self-Disclosure (JSDQ)	0.54	0.83	.06	
Social Desirability (SD)	-0.13	0.09	-.14	
Injury				
Authority	-0.01	0.04	-.02	.08
Restrictiveness	0.07	0.04	.20*	
Disparagement	0.06	0.04	.18	
Self-Disclosure (JSDQ)	0.10	0.22	.04	
Social Desirability (SD)	-0.01	0.02	-.04	

Note. For each dependent variable, the same set of predictors was used. R^2 are for full models. $^*p < .05.$ $^{**}p < .01.$ $^{***}p < .001.$

autonomy and individuality. This complexity may be one reason why there was no significant correlation between Restrictiveness and social desirability. Restrictive partners who show this extreme investment in their partner and their partner's whereabouts may not report high levels of devaluation, although it should be noted that their attitudes are likely to be based on fantasy more than reality and disappointments related to the gap between the two may be one reason violence is high among restrictive partners.

The varying dominance constructs also appeared to have differing associations with varying forms of partner aggression. Restrictiveness emerged as the most important correlate of psychological aggression, physical assault, and injury. Authority demonstrated an inverse association with Negotiation, which may reflect an underlying similarity between the two in that they both refer to decision making in the relationship. Restrictiveness was also associated with the psychologically and physically assaultive behaviors of participants' partners, and, interestingly, Disparagement was also significantly associated with their partner's physical assaults.

Limitations

These findings should be considered preliminary because of two limitations to these data. One, the sample size was smaller than would be desirable. Future psychometric validation of this scale will proceed with enough participants to perform a factor analysis on the entire pool of items. Two, the sample was composed of students, most of whom were in dating relationships. More diverse samples would permit more thorough investigations of differences due to relationship status (married or dating), sex, race, and other factors which may have important associations with dominance.

Implications

These preliminary data suggest that the Dominance Scale is a good operationalization of the new conceptualization of dominance offered in another paper (Hamby, 1996). These early results suggest that distinctions among the different forms are important and can lead to a greater understanding of the ways in which dominance contributes to partner violence.

One important implication of these data is that they provide support for theoretical models which propose that increasing dominance is associated with increasing partner violence. They also suggest a possible reason for the varying results found in studies that use a decision-making measure to assess dominance; this form of dominance, authority, may not be most closely related to partner violence. In this study, the same pattern was found within a single sample that was observed across other published studies: Restrictive control was more related to partner violence than authoritarian control.

The relative symmetry between inflicted and sustained violence is also worthy of note. The similarity between the associations between participants' self-described dominance and both their own and their partners' violence gives an image of an ongoing struggle for control. The fact that participants' disparagement of their partner predicted their partners' violence toward them is also suggestive of ongoing conflict. The association between one's own dominance and sustaining aggression may take several forms. It may be direct, that is, partners of dominant individuals may use aggression to try to break free from the dominating behavior of their partner. Alternatively, the association between one's own dominance and one's partner's aggression may be mediated by one's own violence. In this case, violence by subordinate partners may be self-defensive responses to sustained aggression. Alternatively, both partners may be attempting to be dominant and the resulting violence is multiply and reciprocally determined. Unfortunately, this sample does not include couple data but it would be very interesting to assess the interrelationships of dominance between partners.

Further research to validate these findings is needed, both with the Dominance Scale and with other instruments. Most of the literature on Restrictiveness and Disparagement focuses on courtship violence, including this sample. It will be extremely important to examine whether the same patterns among forms of dominance are found in other samples. As a first step in this direction, the Dominance Scale was distributed to a small sample of female support group members who described their partner's dominance and violence (Bushman & Hamby, 1996). The results showed high internal consistency (.92 to .95) and a similar association among dominance forms and violence to that observed here (albeit with some noteworthy racial differences), offering some corroboration for the findings of this study. Continued study of the dominance construct itself also would be useful, which could be accomplished in part by correlating the Dominance Scale with other measures of dominance in addition to decision making, such as Tolman's (1989) Psychological Maltreatment of Women Inventory. As stated, couple data will also be very important for examining the association between dominance and inflicted and sustained violence. Such issues suggest that further study of dominance is greatly needed, and it is hoped that the Dominance Scale will contribute to future investigations.

REFERENCES

Allen, C. M., & Straus, M. A. (1980). Resources, power, and husband-wife violence. In M. A. Straus & G. T. Hotaling (Eds.), *The social causes of husband-wife violence*. Minneapolis, MN: University of Minnesota Press.

Blood, R. O., & Wolfe, D. M. (1960). *Husbands and wives: The dynamics of married living*. Glencoe, IL: Free Press.

Bruning, J. L., & Kintz, B. L. (1987). *Computational handbook of statistics* (3rd ed.). Glenview, IL: Harper Collins.

Bushman, C. A., & Hamby, S. L. (1996, August). Power, attachment, and partner violence in a female support group sample. In S. L. Hamby (Chair), *Theorizing about gender socialization and power in family violence*. Symposium to be conducted at the 104th annual meeting of the American Psychological Association, Toronto, Ontario.

Campbell, J. C. (1992). Wife-battering: Cultural contexts versus Western social sciences. In D. A. Counts et al. (eds.), *Sanctions and sanctuary: Cultural perspectives on the beating of wives* (pp. 229-250). Boulder, CO: Westview Press.

Coleman, D. H., & Straus, M.A. (1986). Marital power, conflict, and violence in a nationally representative sample of American couples. *Violence and Victims, 1*, 141-157.

Crowne, D. P., & Marlowe, D. (1960). A new scale of social desirability independent of psychopathology. *Journal of Consulting Psychology, 24*, 349-354.

Dobash, R. E., & Dobash, R. P. (1979). *Violence against wives*. New York: The Free Press.

Dutton, D. G. (1994). Patriarchy and wife assault: The ecological fallacy. *Violence and Victims, 9*(2), 167-182.

Dutton, D. G., & Strachan, C. E. (1987). Motivational needs for power and spouse-specific assertiveness in assaultive and nonassaultive men. *Violence and Victims, 2,* 145-156.

Frieze, I. H., & McHugh, M. C. (1992). Power and influence strategies in violent and nonviolent marriages. *Psychology of Women Quarterly, 16,* 449-465.

Fromm, E. (1956). *The art of loving.* New York: Harper & Row.

Gelles, R. J. (1983). An exchange/social control theory. In D. Finkelhor et al. (Eds.), *The dark side of families: Current family violence research* (pp. 151-165). Beverly Hills, CA: Sage.

Goode, W. J. (1971). Force and violence in the family. *Journal of Marriage and the Family, 33,* 624-636.

Gray-Little, B., & Burks, N. (1983). Power and satisfaction in marriage: A review and critique. *Psychological Bulletin, 93,* 513-538.

Haj-Yahia, M. M., & Edleson, J. L. (1994). Predicting the use of conflict resolution tactics among engaged Arab-Palestinian men in Israel. *Journal of Family Violence, 9,* 47-62.

Hamby, S. L. (1992). Women's attitudes towards the use of force in intimate relationships. *Dissertation Abstracts International, 53,* 5976B (Order No. AAC9309886).

Hamby, S. L. (1996). Dominance and its links to partner violence: A typological model. Manuscript in preparation.

Hornung, C. A., McCullough, B. C., & Sugimoto, T. (1981). Status relationship in marriage: Risk factors in spouse abuse. *Journal of Marriage and the Family, 43,* 675-692.

Hotaling, G. T., & Sugarman, D. B. (1986). An analysis of risk markers in husband to wife violence: The current state of knowledge. *Violence and Victims, 1,* 101-124.

Johnson, M. P. (1995). Patriarchal terrorism and common couple violence: Two forms of violence against women. *Journal of Marriage and the Family, 57,* 283-294.

Jourard, S. M. (1971). *Self-disclosure: An experimental analysis of the transparent self.* New York: Wiley.

Koss, M. P., Goodman, L. A., Browne, A., Fitzgerald, L. F., Keita, G. P., & Russo, N. P. (1994). *No safe haven: Male violence against women at home, at work, and in the community.* Washington, DC: American Psychological Association.

Raphael, K. G., & Dohrenwend, B. P. (1987). Self-disclosure and mental health: A problem of confounded measurement. *Journal of Abnormal Psychology, 96,* 214-217.

Rouse, L. P. (1990). The dominance motive in abusive partners: Identifying couples at risk. *Journal of College Student Development, 31,* 330-335.

Spitzberg, B. H., & Marshall, L. L. (1991, May). *Courtship violence and relational outcomes*. Presented at the International Communication Association Conference, Chicago, IL.

Stets, J. E. (1992). Interactive processes in dating aggression: A national study. *Journal of Marriage and the Family, 54,* 165-177.

Stets, J. E., & Pirog-Good, M. A. (1990). Interpersonal control and courtship aggression. *Journal of Social and Personal Relationships, 7,* 371-394.

Straus, M. A., Hamby, S. L., Boney-McCoy, S., & Sugarman, D. B. (1996). The Revised Conflicts Tactics Scales (CTS2): Development and preliminary psychometric data. *Journal of Family Issues, 17,* 283-316.

Tolman, R. M. (1989). The development of a measure of psychological treatment of women by their male partner. *Violence and Victims, 4,* 159-177.

Wills, T. A. (1981). Downward comparison principles in social psychology. *Psychological Bulletin, 90,* 245-271.

Yllö, K. (1984). The status of women, marital equality, and violence against wives. *Journal of Family Issues, 5,* 307-320.

Yllö, K., & Bograd, M. (1988). *Feminist perspectives on wife abuse*. Newbury Park, CA: Sage.

APPENDIX

The Dominance Scale

People have many different ways of relating to each other. The following statements are all different ways of relating to or thinking about your partner. Please read each statement and decide how much you agree with it.

4 = Strongly Agree
3 = Agree
2 = Disagree
1 = Strongly Disagree

1) My partner often has good ideas.
2) I try to keep my partner from spending time with opposite sex friends.
3) If my partner and I can't agree, I usually have the final say.
4) It bothers me when my partner makes plans without talking to me first.
5) My partner doesn't have enough sense to make important decisions.
6) I hate losing arguments with my partner.
7) My partner should not keep any secrets from me.
8) I insist on knowing where my partner is at all times.
9) When my partner and I watch TV, I hold the remote control.
10) My partner and I generally have equal say about decisions.
11) It would bother me if my partner made more money than I did.

12) I generally consider my partner's interests as much as mine.

13) I tend to be jealous.

14) Things are easier in my relationship if I am in charge.

15) Sometimes I have to remind my partner of who's boss.

16) 1 have a right to know everything my partner does.

17) It would make me mad if my partner did something I had said not to do.

18) Both partners in a relationship should have equal say about decisions.

19) If my partner and I can't agree. I should have the final say.

20) I understand there are some things my partner may not want to talk about with me.

21) My partner needs to remember that I am in charge.

22) My partner is a talented person.

23) It's hard for my partner to learn new things.

24) People usually like my partner.

25) My partner makes a lot of mistakes.

26) My partner can handle most things that happen.

27) I sometimes think my partner is unattractive.

28) My partner is basically a good person.

29) My partner doesn't know how to act in public.

30) I often tell my partner how to do something.

31) I dominate my partner.

32) I have a right to be involved with anything my partner does.

Chapter 5

A Scale for Identifying "Stockholm Syndrome" Reactions in Young Dating Women: Factor Structure, Reliability, and Validity

Dee L. R. Graham, Edna I. Rawlings, Kim Ihms, Diane Latimer, Janet Foliano, Alicia Thompson, Kelly Suttman, Mary Farrington, and Rachel Hacker

D rawing on the literatures of nine different "hostage" groups, Graham developed the Stockholm Syndrome theory to explain certain paradoxical behaviors commonly observed in these groups. These paradoxes include professing "love" for persons who abuse them, defending their abusers even after severe beatings, blaming themselves for the abuse done to them, and denying or minimizing the threatening nature of the abuse.

The psychodynamics of the Stockholm Syndrome (also referred to as "traumatic bonding" [Dutton & Painter, 1981] and "terror bonding" [Barry, 1995]), as described by Graham (1994), involve hostages/victims experiencing a threat to their survival while, if kindness is perceived, developing hope that they will be permitted to live. Under these conditions, and if no other avenue of escape is perceived, the frightened victims deny both their terror and the captor's abuse and *bond* to the kind side of the captor, who represents their only available source of succor and avenue for escaping abuse. Thus, according to Graham (1994), four necessary *precursors* of the syndrome are: (a) the victim perceiving a threat to his or her survival; (b) the victim perceiving some kindness, however small, from the abuser/captor; (c) the victim being isolated from others who might offer an alternative perspective from that of the abuser; and (d) the victim perceiving no way to escape except by winning over the abuser. Numerous cognitive and perceptual distortions develop as a defense against terror, including denial, rationalization, and minimization of abuse. From the nine hostage literatures reviewed, Graham identified 66 *aspects* (behavior, attitudes, and beliefs) potentially associated with this syndrome. For a list of these aspects, see Graham (1994).

In addition, Graham proposed that coping with prolonged, severe threat to survival causes the victim/captive to internalize the captor-captive dynamics and to generalize them to relations with others. This generalization (of survival strategies developed in interaction with the abuser/captor) results in changes in interpersonal functioning that include (a) splitting, (b) displaced rage, (c) intense push-pull dynamics, and (d) loss of sense of self. Because these four long-term outcomes of Stockholm Syndrome also characterize borderline personality disorder (BPD), Graham and Rawlings (1991) hypothesized that BPD could be produced, even in adults, by chronic interpersonal abuse.

Others positing a posttraumatic stress theory of the etiology of BPD—for example, Barnard and Hirsch (1985), Herman and van der Kolk (1987), Lipari (1992), and Westen, Ludolph, Misle, Ruffins, and Block (1990)—have obtained empirical support for the argument that BPD is produced by chronic, recurrent *childhood* trauma. Brende (1983) and Lindy (1988) observed BPD-like symptoms in Vietnam veterans exposed to *trauma in adulthood*. It is likely that prolonged trauma experienced in adulthood produces BPD symptoms that are less severe and shorter term than that experienced in childhood, though observations suggest a similar constellation of symptoms may be produced regardless of the age of victims. For this reason, Graham (1994) has proposed that victims of abuse fall along a continuum of interpersonal functioning, described at one end by no BPD characteristics and no generalization and, at the other end, by BPD and generalization of abuser-victim dynamics. Walker and Brown (Brown, 1992) and Herman (1992) have independently proposed similar diagnostic schemes for victims of chronic interpersonal abuse that would encompass the borderline continuum described by Graham (1994).

THE TRAUMATIC BONDING THEORY
OF DUTTON AND PAINTER

Dutton and Painter's (1993) theory of traumatic bonding is similar in some ways to Graham's Stockholm Syndrome theory. According to these theorists, strong emotional attachments are formed in relationships characterized by two factors: power imbalance and intermittent good-bad treatment The power imbalance creates a power dynamic in which both the subordinate and dominant partner become increasingly dependent on each other. In battering relationships, physical and emotional abuse by the dominant partner serves to create and maintain the power imbalance. The alternation of reinforcement and punishment produces the powerful emotional bonding of the victim to the abuser. According to these authors, this emotional bond interferes with detaching from, leaving, or remaining outside of an abusive relationship. They liken this emotional bond to an "elastic band which stretches away from the abuser with time and subsequently 'snaps' the woman back" (p. 109). With time away from the abuser, these authors expect that memory of past abuse fades and fear subsides. At such a time, "the strength of the traumatically-formed bond reveals itself through an incremental focus on the desirable aspects of the relationship, and a subsequent sudden and dramatic shift in the woman's 'belief gestalt' about the relationship" (p. 110).

RELATION OF LOVE TO COPING
FOLLOWING VIOLENCE

Graham (1994) has hypothesized that cognitive distortions such as denial, minimization, and rationalization of abuse are critical components of the psychodynamics of bonding with an abuser. Rationalization is seen in victims who, for example, describe the violence inflicted on them by their partners as "justified." Sigelman, Berry, and Wiles (1984) discovered that among the victims of dating violence, 43% felt that their partner's violence was at least "somewhat justified." Minimization of violence was seen in a study by O'Keeffe, Broackopp, and Chew (1986). These researchers found that only 21% of victims felt that violence hurt their relationship, 30% felt that it had no effect, and 21% reported that it actually improved their relationship. Only 12% ended the relationship because of the violence.

Cognitive confusion of emotions may occur in victims of violence where physiological arousal caused by fear is interpreted as attraction (cf. Walster, 1971). By engaging in cognitive distortions—such as convincing themselves that violence either has not hurt or has actually improved their relationships or that violence is evidence of love—victims may be able to create a bond, maintain a bond, or bond more strongly with an abusive partner.

Koval and Lloyd (1986; cited by Lo & Sporakowski, 1989) found that individuals who remained in violent dating relationships, as compared with those who left; both had more commitment and loved their partners more. Similar findings were obtained by Follingstad, Rutledge, Polek, and McNeill-Hawkins (1988). Lo and Sporakowski (1989) found that a majority (77%) of dating couples who reported relationship violence planned to continue in the relationship. The reasons they gave for continuing were love and enjoying dating their partners.

Flynn (1990) studied a sample of 59 college women who felt they had been victimized in a noncohabiting, dating relationship and who ended the relationship, at least in part because of the partners' violence against them. After the first violent episode, only 7 women immediately ended the relationship. Fifty percent of the women stayed with the partner for 3 months after the first episode of violence. The amount of love women felt for their partners correlated positively with both length of stay following abuse ($r = .52$) and frequency of violence ($r = .38$). Multiple regression revealed that the number of days the women stayed with their partners following the partners' first use of violence against them *increased* when: violence was more frequent, the women felt more love, and the couple had been dating for a longer time before the violence occurred. The single best predictor of length of stay following abuse was frequency of violence, suggesting that more frequent violence was associated with reductions in possible avenues of escape for the women. This interpretation is supported by Follingstad and colleagues' (1988) finding that women who remained in ongoing physically violent relationships had partners who were more controlling than women who left after the first incident of physical violence.[2] If our interpretation is correct, the women may have coped with perceived inescapable violence by traumatically bonding with their abusers, as indicated by their reports of feeling more love the greater the violence experienced. The women's reported commitment and "love" may have been cognitive distortions that functioned both to reduce the women's terror and to enable the development of a *mutual* bond between abuser and victim. This explanation provides one account—a Stockholm Syndrome theory account—for why violent relationships would be experienced as more intimate than nonviolent ones.[3]

A research study conducted by Dutton and Painter (1993) of abused women separated from their partners showed that, immediately following separation and 6 months after, intermittency of abuse (that is, the negativeness of negative behaviors *during* abuse plus the positiveness of positive behaviors *after* the abuse) and power shifts resulting from batterings were the best predictors of an abuse syndrome composed of three significantly related dependent variables: attachment, lowered self-esteem, and experienced trauma. Women with the lowest self-esteem had experienced the most trauma and were the most attached. At 6 months following separation, as compared to immediately following separation, although only 9% of the women had returned to live with their abusers, there were no changes in self-esteem, 73% of attachment scores were as strong, and experienced trauma scores were 57% lower.

In sum, evidence indicates that, for many women, abuse is positively associated with both strength of attachment and longevity of relationship following abuse. Even after separating from abusive partners, victims frequently remain strongly attached to them. According to the Stockholm Syndrome theory, this paradoxical attachment is a strategy for both coping with and ending that abuse.

ASSESSING STOCKHOLM SYNDROME IN DATING RELATIONSHIPS

In order to test Graham's Stockholm Syndrome theory, it was first necessary to develop a psychometrically sound instrument to measure the syndrome. Because the present researchers function in a college setting and our interest was in helping therapists identify young women who show the syndrome in relations with abusive dating partners, we decided to develop an instrument on a sample of young college women in heterosexual dating relationships.

Are dating relationships sufficiently violent for one to expect to find evidence of Stockholm Syndrome? In a national sample of about 2,600 college women, White and Koss (1991) found that approximately 35% had sustained some type of physical violence and 87% to 88% had sustained some form of psychological violence. In another national sample composed of 3,187 college women, Koss, Gidycz, and Wisniewski (1987) found that 57% of women had experienced some form of sexual victimization, with 15.4% having experienced rape. Thus, almost all college women suffer some form of violence— especially psychological violence—in at least one dating relationship. Even if violence in dating relationships is mutually inflicted by male and female partners, as White and Koss's (1991) data suggest, one would expect Stockholm Syndrome dynamics to be present in female/male dating relationships due to the patriarchal nature of Western culture. For example, young men are expected to choose female dating partners who are smaller and less strong, and who have less power than them (Graham, 1994). For these reasons, women are more likely than men to fear their partners, suffer injuries, and develop psychosomatic symptoms.

The purposes of the following studies were both to determine, for a college dating sample, the factor structure of a Stockholm Syndrome scale that would be suitable for use in future studies of dating violence and to assess the reliability and validity of the scale and its emergent subscales.

Measurement Issues

STUDY 1: FACTOR STRUCTURE

The purpose of Study 1 was to identify the factor structure of the Stockholm Syndrome scale for women in dating relationships and to begin to assess its concurrent validity. For the latter purpose, scales measuring trauma and BPD characteristics were used. The Stockholm Syndrome scale was expected to correlate positively with both. The correlation of the scale with social desirability was also assessed.

Method

Subjects. The sample was composed of 764 undergraduate women from the Introduction to Psychology Subject Pool at the University of Cincinnati.

Procedure. Participation involved completion of a 392-item questionnaire, requiring approximately $1^{1}/_{2}$ hours; however, only 208 of the first 245 items were analyzed for the purposes of the present study. Findings regarding the remaining 184 items will be reported elsewhere.

Questionnaire. The questionnaire consisted of five parts: (a) 33 demographic and relationship background questions, (b) a 127-item Stockholm Syndrome scale, (c) the 15- item Impact of Event Scale (Horowitz, Wilner, & Alvarez, 1979), (d) the 18-item Borderline Personality Disorder scale (BPD scale) of the Personality Diagnostic Questionnaire (Hyler & Rieder, 1987), and (e) a 15-item short form of the Marlowe-Crowne Social Desirability scale (Crowne & Marlowe, 1960). Because victims of abuse often do not recognize that they have been abused, the word "abuse" was avoided throughout the questionnaire. Descriptions of specific behaviors—that are abusive but were not labeled as such—or the phrases, "when my partner is really angry at me," and "when my partner has gotten so angry at me that he has hurt my feelings," were used in place of the word "abuse."

Graham, Rawlings, and associates wrote one or more items per aspect to assess each of the 66 potential Stockholm Syndrome aspects in a dating sample. These aspects, stated in the language of captive/hostage relations, assessed both feelings and actions. An example of an aspect and the items measuring it are:

> Aspect: "Captive shows splitting."
> Items: "I switch back and forth between seeing my partner as either all good or all bad."
> "I tend to see my partner as good and me as bad."

Most aspects were composed of only two items. Items were written in terms of "I," "me," and "partner" and not in terms of "captive" and "captor." All items and scale scores ranged from 0 ("never or almost never" or "not applicable") to 4 ("always or almost always"), with 4 representing a greater degree of the syndrome.

The Impact of Event Scale (IES; Horowitz et al., 1979) is a self-report measure that is designed to assess responses to stressful life events, or trauma. Because abuse in dating relationships is often chronic rather than acute, the stressful life event assessed in the current study was "times that my partner has gotten really angry at me." Horowitz and colleagues (1979) reported the split-half reliability to be .86. Test-retest reliability was .87 for the total scale.

BPD characteristics were measured using Hyler and Rieder's (1987) BPD scale, developed to assess DSM-III-R criteria for the diagnosis of BPD. The validity of the scale was supported by Hyler, Skodol, Kellman, Oldham, and Rosnick's (1990) finding that it significantly agreed with both the Personality Disorder Examination and the Structured Clinical Interview for DSM-III-R Personality Disorders, two structured interview instruments, in diagnosing BPD in a clinical sample. In the current study, scores for the BPD scale were positively skewed, a condition that was corrected through use of a square root transformation m all subsequent analyses.

A 15-item short form of the Marlowe-Crowne Social Desirability scale (M-C SDS; Crowne & Marlowe, 1960) was used. The 15 items were randomly selected from the original 33-item scale. The greater the number of items endorsed on this scale, the more a respondent is thought to be "faking good" or trying to present herself in a favorable manner.

Results

Demographics. The sample was composed of undergraduates, primarily of first-year students (63.6%) or sophomores (24.9%). Ages ranged from 17 to 38 with a median age of 19.0 years. Partners' ages ranged from 16 to 40 with a median age of 20.0 years. The sample was predominantly White (87.0%), with some African-American (10.1%) and Asian (2.5%) women. It was also predominantly Catholic (43.8%), with 22.4% Protestant. Although 70.8% of the women were employed, most (71.4%) had annual incomes below $4,000. Most of their partners' incomes were below $4,999 (55.0%). Most women lived either in their family's home (41.7%) or a college dormitory (36.1%). Only 2.7% were currently living with a partner.

Although 60.7% of the female students were dating only this partner, and an additional 6.9% were engaged to him, 27.1 % were dating this partner plus others. For most, the length of their relationship with their partner was either 1 to 6 months (29.8%),7 months to 1 year (26.0%), or 2 to 3 years (32.1%). Although 4.8% were currently separated from their partner, 44.3% had broken up with him one or more times.

Item Relevance. No items were answered by fewer than 99% of the sample. An item was omitted from analysis if its endorsement rate was 15% or less, that is, if 15% or less of the sample answered "seldom" or more often than seldom in response to it. Eight of the 127 items fell below this criterion and were omitted from the factor analysis.

Stockholm Syndrome Factors. Kaiser's Measure of Sampling Adequacy was .95 for the overall scale and ranged from .87 to .98 for individual items. An iterated principal factor solution, in which prior communality estimates for variables were set to their maximum absolute correlation with any other variable, identified 10 factors with eigen values greater than 1. Examination of the scree plot from the iterated principal factors analysis revealed either Three or four factors. Both iterated principal factor solutions (three and four factors) were examined, using varimax rotation of the factors. A four-factor solution was found to be the most theoretically meaningful. The variance explained by each of the factors was: Factor 1, 37.36%; Factor 2, 30.14%; Factor 3, 23.08%; and Factor 4, 9.41%. Only items that loaded .50 or greater were retained in a subscale. No items loading on the fourth factor met the .50 criterion. The resulting scale with its three subscales is presented in Table 1, with the factor on which each item loaded and its loading on that factor shown in parentheses. These three factors accounted for 67.0% of the common variance pool. Iterated principal factor solutions and common factor analysis yielded virtually identical subscales when a varimax rotation was performed.[4]

Names and Characterizations of the Stockholm Syndrome Factors. The three factors were named Core Stockholm Syndrome (Factor 1), Psychological Damage (Factor 2), and Love-Dependence (Factor 3) for reasons that follow. These reasons are not listed in their order of importance.

Factor 1 was named *Core Stockholm Syndrome* because it was composed of items suggestive of: (a) interpersonal *trauma* (e.g., 11, 34, 42, 23, and 22); (b) *cognitive distortions* central to Stockholm Syndrome (rationalization of the partner's angry behavior, Items 7, 14, and 38; self-blame for the partner's angry behavior, Items 3, 8, 26, and 27; siding with partner against others, Items 37 and 40; projection of one's victim status onto the abuser, Items 7, 17, and 21 [cf. Hacker, 1976]); and (c) other adaptations observed to occur in hostages with Stockholm Syndrome (e.g., hope created by small kindnesses, Items 30 and 43, and, most notably, the presence of love in the context of fear and the belief that love may stop the partner from getting angry, Items 20 and 12). In sum, this factor appeared to measure the use of strategies for coping with interpersonal abuse.

Factor 2, named *Psychological Damage,* was composed of items indicative of depression (35 and 41), low self-esteem (32 [reverse coded] and 48), loss of sense of self (18, 25, 39, 44, 45, and 46), and interpersonal difficulties (9). Many of these items (9, 18, 25, 39, 44, 45, 46, and 48) suggest BPD characteristics.

Factor 3 was named *Love-Dependence* because its items (2 and 4) revealed that an endorser believed that her survival was dependent on her partner's love. In addition, the endorser was "extremely attached" to her partner (Item 5),

**TABLE 1. The Stockholm Syndrome Scale, Factors
on Which Each Item Loaded, and the Items' Factor Loadings[a]**

Using the letters,
  A. I always or almost always feel this way
  B. I often feel this way
  C. I feel this way as often as not
  D. I seldom feel this way
  E. I never or almost never feel this way; this does not apply to me,
indicate the extent to which each of the statements below describes how you feel or
have felt *since being with your partner*:
  1. My partner's love and protection are more important than any hurt he might cause me. (Love, .50)
  2. I need my partner's nurturance and protection to survive. (Love, .73)
  3. The problem is not that my partner is "just an angry person"; it is that I provoke him. (Core, .57)
  4. I have to have my partner's love to survive. (Love, .78)
  5. I am extremely attached to my partner. (Love, .64)
  6. In my eyes, my partner is like a god. (Love, .57)
  7. My partner would not get so angry at me if others had not been mean to him. (Core, .54)
  8. There is something about me that makes my partner unable to control his anger. (Core, .61)
  9. When I start getting close to people, something bad happens. (Damage, .53)
  10. Other people see only my partner's negative side; they don't see all the small kindnesses he does for me that make me love him. (Core, .50)
  11. I do not want others to know how angry my partner gets at me. (Core, .64)
  12. I both love and fear my partner. (Core, .65)
  13. I dislike others telling me my partner is not good to me. (Core, .5?)
  14. I know my partner is not a violent person; he just loses control. (Core, .58)
  15. Without my partner, I have nothing to live for. (Love, .70)
  16. I feel like I am going crazy. (Damage, .52)
  17. My partner is like me, a victim of others' anger. (Core, .50)
  18. I do not know who I am. (Damage, .68)
  19. I cannot imagine trying to live without my partner. (Love, .77)
  20. If I give my partner enough love, he will stop getting so angry at me. (Core, .71)
  21. My partner is as much a victim as I am. (Core, .61)
  22. I have conflicting feelings about my partner. (Core, .50)
  23. It is really hard for me to question whether my relationship with my partner is good for me. (Core, .50)
  24. If my relationship were to break up, I would feel so much pain that I would want to kill myself. (Love, .62)
  25. I cannot stand it if I even suspect somebody is rejecting me in any way. (Damage, .52)
  26. I hate those parts of me that cause my partner to criticize or get angry at me. (Core, .52)

Continued

TABLE 1. (Continued)

Using the letters,
  A. Always or almost always
  B. Often
  C. As often as not
  D. Seldom
  E. Almost never or never,
indicate the extent to which you do or have done the following *since being with your partner:*

27. Because I cause my partner to get angry at me, I am not a good partner. (Core, .50)
28. The more I talk to people, the more confused I get about whether my relationship with my partner is healthy. (Core, .59)
29. Without my partner, I would not know who I am. (Love, .55)
30. Any kindness by my partner creates hope in me that things will get better. (Core, .52)
31. I feel good about who I am. (Damage, .63; reverse coded)
32. I feel calm and sure of myself. (Damage, .66; reverse coded)
33. Aspects of my partner's and my relationship that I see as normal, others see as unhealthy. (Core, .53)
34. There are things that my partner has done to me that I don't like to think about. (Core, .56)
35. I feel down and blue. (Damage, .68)
36. I feel like I could not live without my partner. (Love, .73)
37. If others try to intervene on my behalf when my partner criticizes me or gets angry with me, I take my partner's side against them. (Core, .54)
38. I find myself defending and making excuses for my partner when I talk about him with others. (Core, .57)
39. When others ask me how I feel about something, I do not know. (Damage, .56)
40. If others try to intervene on my behalf when my partner criticizes me, I get angry at them. (Core, .53)
41. I find it difficult to concentrate on tasks. (Damage, .60)
42. I switch back and forth between seeing my partner as either all good or all bad. (Core, .54)
43. When my partner is less critical of me, I become hopeful. (Core, 50)
44. It is hard for me to make decisions. (Damage, .55)
45. I have different personalities depending on who I am with. (Damage, .52)
46. I cannot make decisions. (Damage, .61)
47. I make jokes to others about the times my partner has been really angry at me. (Core, .57)
48. I work hard to get people to like me. (Damage, .52)
49. I get angry at people who point out ways in which my partner is not good to me. (Core, .50)

[a]The factor on which each item loaded and the factor loading for that item are indicated in parentheses.   Core = Core Stockholm Syndrome;
Damage = Psychological Damage; Love = Love-Dependence.

idolized him (Item 6), and believed that her partner's love and protection were more important than any pain he might cause her (Item 1). She also felt that, without her partner, she would not know who she was (Item 29), would have nothing to live for (Item 15), could not live (Item 36), and would want to kill herself (Item 2). Perhaps for these reasons, she could not imagine trying to live without her partner (Item 19).

Scale and Subscale Definitions. For all three subscales, subscale scores calculated by equally weighting all the items comprising a subscale correlated at least .99 with subscale scores calculated by weighting each item using its factor loading. For this reason, all subsequent analyses utilized subscale scores that were the mean of women's scores on all the items comprising a subscale, with each item weighted equally (namely, x1).

Three alternative ways of defining the overall scale were examined: (a) as the mean of women's three subscale scores; (b) as a weighted sum of women's subscale scores, using the variance explained by each factor as a weight, and (c) as the sum of women's scores for all items comprising the three subscales. Definition *a* correlated with definitions *b* and *c* .99 and .98, respectively. Definition *b* correlated with definition *c* .99. Definition *a* was used hereafter.

Internal Consistency of Scale and Subscales. Cronbach alphas were .94 for Core Stockholm Syndrome, .90 for Psychological Damage, and .89 for Love-Dependence. Using uncorrected correlations, the subscales correlated as follows with the overall scale: Core Stockholm Syndrome, .80; Psychological Damage, .82; and Love-Dependence, .74.

Scale's and Subscales' Distribution Characteristics. The average endorsement rate of the 49 items comprising the three subscales was 47.42%, indicating that, on the average, approximately half the women endorsed any given scale item. The scores for all subscales were significantly positively skewed. Thus, although women's scores ranged from 0 to 3.462 for both Core Stockholm Syndrome and Psychological Damage and from 0 to 3.600 for Love-Dependence (subscale scores potentially ranged from 0 to 4), mean scores for the three subscales were low. The means and standard deviations were: overall scale, .857 (SD = .552); Core Stockholm Syndrome, .697 (SD = .586); Psychological Damage, 1.008 (SD = .698); and Love-Dependence, .976 (SD = .800). These mean scores indicate women "seldom" felt or did what the Stockholm Syndrome items asked about, and thus suggest that the scale might function better for an abused clinical sample than for a nonclinical one. Despite this floor effect, standard deviations tended to be high, indicating a fair amount of variability in women's responses to subscale items.

Relation of Stockholm Syndrome to Demographics and Relationship Variables. One-way analysis of variance (ANOVA) was utilized to assess the relationship of the overall scale to demographic and relationship variables. Due to the fact that the subscales' scores were positively skewed, multivariate analysis of variance (MANOVA) was not used to assess the relationship of the subscale scores to these same variables. Transformation of scale and subscale scores was considered and rejected due to a desire to maintain the interpretability of scale scores. Fortunately, ANOVA is robust as regards the assumption of normality, particularly when sample sizes are large. ANOVA results are shown in Table 2.

Overall Stockholm Syndrome did not differ as a function of religion; however, it differed by race, $F(2,759) = 3.92$, $p = .02$. Scheffe' tests revealed that Black women reported less of the syndrome than did White women ($p < .05$), and would most likely have reported less than Asian women had the number of Asians included in the study been higher.

One would expect more Stockholm Syndrome to be evidenced in serious, or long-term, relationships than in newly formed ones. This expectation was supported. The syndrome differed as a function of length of relationship, with those women who had dated their partners for 6 months or shorter reporting less of the syndrome than those who had dated their partners for longer, $F(1,762) = 26.56$, $p < .00005$.

Separations (breakups) are an indication of distress in the relationship. Thus, one would expect higher Stockholm Syndrome among women who were separated from their partners than among those who were not. Furthermore, the more separations women had experienced from their partners, the higher one would expect their Stockholm Syndrome to be. Again, both expectations were affirmed. Overall Stockholm Syndrome differed as a function of relationship status, $F(3,762) = 5.53$, $p < .01$. Scheffe' tests revealed that women who were currently separated from their partners evidenced more of the syndrome than did women who were dating either the partner only or the partner as well as others ($p < .05$). In addition, women's overall Stockholm Syndrome differed as a function of the number of times the couple had separated, $F(4,761) = 11.43$, $p < .00005$. Scheffe' tests revealed that women who had experienced no or one separation from their partners reported less of the syndrome than did those who had experienced two or four separations ($p < .05$).

Having a partner become so angry that he hurt one's feelings is another possible sign of a distressed relationship. Potentially, such behavior is a form of psychological abuse. One would expect, then, both that having a partner behave this way would be associated with Stockholm Syndrome, and that the more times this behavior was exhibited, the higher a woman's Stockholm Syndrome would be. Both expectations were confirmed. Women who had noticed their partner behaving this way, as compared to those who had not, reported significantly higher Stockholm Syndrome, $F(1,762) = 120.22$, $p < .00005$. Also, the number of times a partner had been this angry was related to women's overall Stockholm Syndrome, $F(4,762) = 31.91$, $p < .00005$. Scheffe' tests showed that women who had never had their partners express anger in this fashion reported less Stockholm Syndrome than those who *had* noticed it occurring ($p < .05$), and women who had noticed it occurring only

TABLE 2. Relation of Overall Stockholm Syndrome to Demographics and Relationship Variables

Item	N	Mean	F	df	p
Relationship status			5.53	3,762	.0009
Dating P + others	207	.83[a]			
Dating P only	463	.83[b]			
Separated	40	1.18[a,b]			
Engaged	53	.94			
Race			3.92	2,759	.0202
Black	77	.70a			
White	664	.87a			
Asian	19	1.01			
Religion			.66	4,762	ns
Catholic	334	.88			
Protestant	171	.80			
Jewish	21	.82			
Other	157	.87			
None	79	.84			
Length of relationship			26.56	1,762	<.00005
≤ 6 months	279	.72			
≥ 7 months	484	.93			
Number of separations			11.43	4,761	<.00005
None	425	.77[a,b]			
1	90	.86[c,d]			
2	75	1.09[a-c]			
3	32	.90			
≥4	40	1.24[b,d]			
Ever noticed *P* sometimes gets so angry at you that he hurts your feelings?			120.22	1,762	<.00005
No	381	.65			
Yes	382	1.06			
Number of times *P* has been this angry at you?			31.91	4,762	<.00005
Never	324	.66[a,b,c,d]			
1-2 times	184	.83[a,e,f,g]			
3-5 times	152	1. 08[b,e]			
6-10 times	48	1.21[c,f]			
≥ 11 times	55	1.19[d,g]			

Note. For each item, means with superscripts of the same letter differ significantly, as indicated by Scheffe' tests.

P = partner.

once or twice reported less Stockholm Syndrome than those who had witnessed its occurrence on three or more occasions ($p < .05$).

   Social Desirability and Concurrent Validity. Correlations between Stockholm Syndrome and the IES, the BPD scale, and the M-C SDS are presented in Table 3 (Study 1). Core Stockholm Syndrome and Psychological Damage were fairly highly correlated ($r = .65$). The higher a woman scored on Social Desirability, the lower she scored on the Stockholm Syndrome scale and each of its subscales; this was particularly the case for Psychological Damage ($r = -.39$). The correlation of Love-Dependence with the M-C SDS was significant only because of the large number of respondents on which the analysis was performed and may not be meaningful.

   Also shown in Table 3 (Study 1), the scale and all three of its subscales correlated positively and significantly with both BPD and IES scores, although the correlation of Love-Dependence with BPD was so low as to possibly not be meaningful. The IES correlated most highly with Core Stockholm Syndrome ($r = .82$). The BPD scale correlated highest with Psychological Damage ($r = .48$).[5]

STUDY 2: TEST-RETEST RELIABILITY

The purpose of this study was to assess the test-retest reliability of the Stockholm Syndrome scale and each of its factors.

TABLE 3. Correlations of Stockholm Syndrome Scale and Factors With Each Other and With the Marlowe-Crowne Social Desirability Scale, Horowitz, Wilner, and Alvarez' Impact of Event Scale, Hyler and Rieder's Borderline Personality Disorder Scale, Straus' Conflict Tactics Scales,[a] and Hatfield and Sprecher's Passionate Love Scale

Scale	Study 1 ($n = 763$)					Study 3 ($n = 278$)			
	Damage	Love	M-C SDS	IES	BPD[b]	Reason	PsyViol	PhViol[b]	PLS
Core[c]	.65*	.33*	-.24*	.82*	.38*	.03	.55*	.34*	.25*
Damage		.32*	-.39*	.54*	.48*	-.04	.30*	.17*	.27*
Love			-.14*	.36*	.17*	.03	.28*	.13*	.62*
SS			-.32*	.70*	.42*	.02	.46*	.26*	.48*

[a]Straus' Verbal Aggression scale is here called Psychological Violence. His Violence scale is here called Physical Violence. [b]A square root transformation was performed on women's BPD and Physical Violence scores. [c]Core = Core Stockholm Syndrome; Damage = Psychological Damage; Love = Love-Dependence; SS = Stockholm Syndrome; M-C SDS = Marlowe-Crowne Social Desirability scale; IES = Impact of Event Scale; BPD = Borderline Personality Disorder Scale; PsyViol = Psychological Violence; PhViol = Physical Violence; PLS = Passionate Love Scale.
* $p < .05$ (two-tailed).

Method

The new 49-item Stockholm Syndrome scale, resulting from the factor analysis performed in Study 1, was administered to a new nonclinical sample of 123 undergraduate women in dating relationships who were members of the Introduction to Psychology Subject Pool. The women were asked to complete the same questionnaire on two occasions, 2 weeks apart. Only 108 women both returned to take the scale a second time and had complete data sets.

Results

The demographics of this sample approximated those described in Study 1. The *t* tests for independent samples revealed that the 15 subjects who failed to retake the questionnaire did not differ significantly from the 108 women who returned for retesting on either the overall scale or any of its subscales. The 2-week test-retest reliabilities were .84 for the overall scale, .85 for Core Stockholm Syndrome, .81 for Psychological Damage, and .78 for Love-Dependence ($n = 108$).

The *t* tests for correlated groups indicated that women's overall scale scores and Love-Dependence scores were significantly higher upon initial testing than upon retesting: overall scale, .83 vs. .75, $t(107) = 2.93$, $p = .004$; Love-Dependence, .85 vs. .70, $t(107) = 3.32$, $p = .001$). A nonsignificant trend in that direction was found for Core Stockholm Syndrome, .66 vs. .60; $t(107) = 1.89$, $p = .06$. Psychological Damage scores were in the same, albeit nonsignificant, direction.

STUDY 3: CONCURRENT VALIDITY

If Stockholm Syndrome represents a response to violence, then one would expect the three Stockholm Syndrome subscales both to correlate positively with partners' use of psychological and/or physical violence and to show no relation to partners' use of civil discourse, or discourse void of violence. Straus' (1979) Conflict Tactics Scales assess all three dimensions: psychological violence (the Verbal Aggression scale), physical violence (the Violence scale), and reasoning, respectively.[6]

The purpose of this study was to assess the concurrent validity of the Stockholm Syndrome scale and its factors using Straus' three scales. Also, because Stockholm Syndrome represents a response to trauma that involves bonding with one's captor or abuser, the authors sought to assess the correlation of the Stockholm Syndrome scale with a measure of love, namely, Hatfield and Sprecher's (1986) Passionate Love Scale. It was hypothesized that the Stockholm Syndrome scale would correlate positively with both the Passionate Love Scale and Straus' Psychological and Physical Violence scales, but not Straus' Reasoning scale.

Method

The sample, composed of 278 undergraduate women, was administered a questionnaire consisting of the 49-item Stockholm Syndrome scale, Straus' (1979) 18-item Conflict Tactics Scale (CTS), Form N, and Hatfield and Sprecher's (1986) 30-item Passionate Love Scale (PLS).

Using the CTS, the women were asked to indicate how many times in the past 12 months their partners had used each of 18 different conflict tactics— ranging from discussing an issue calmly to using a knife or a gun—during a conflict or disagreement. Although "cried" was one of the 18 items comprising the CTS, it was not included in the definitions of any of the subscales (cf., Straus, 1979). The response scale was modified to read: "never," "once,'" "twice," "3–5 times," and "6 or more times."

The CTS is the most frequently used measure of violence in relationships. Straus (1979) reports findings supporting the internal consistency and the concurrent validity of the CTS. (See also Schumm & Bagarozzi [1989].) Arias and Beach (1987) found that reports of partner's aggressive behavior were not affected by social desirability. Because the Physical Violence scale scores were highly skewed, a square root transformation was performed on them in the correctional analyses to follow.

Although Hatfield and Sprecher (1986) used a 9-point response scale with the PLS, a 5- point response scale was used in the current study. Also, whereas Hatfield and Sprecher leave a blank in each item and ask the respondent to "think of the person whom you love most passionately *right now*, " we inserted the words "my partner," thereby making the language of the scale consistent with the rest of the questionnaire. Hatfield and Sprecher found the PLS to be unidimensional, highly internally consistent, uncorrelated with social desir- ability, and highly correlated with other measures of intimacy. Research by Hendrick and Hendrick (1989) has also provided support for the concurrent validity of the PLS.

Results

Correlations between the Stockholm Syndrome scale, its subscales, and both the CTS and the PLS are shown in Table 3 (Study 3). As expected, the Stockholm Syndrome scale correlated significantly and positively with both Straus' Psychological and Physical Violence scales and nonsignificantly with his Reasoning scale. Similar findings were obtained between the Stockholm Syndrome subscales and the CTS. Also as expected, the Stockholm Syndrome scale correlated significantly and positively with the PLS, as did the scale's three subscales, with Love-Dependence correlating the most highly with the PLS ($r = .61$).

DISCUSSION

Three strong factors emerged upon factor analysis of the 119-item Stockholm Syndrome scale. The three subscales created from these factors—comprising a total of 49 items— showed excellent internal consistency and good test-retest reliability. Amazingly, the three subscales that emerged were conceptually similar to the three variables that Dutton and Painter (1993) concluded "constitute a syndrome of interrelated effects of abuse" (p. 116): attachment, lowered self-esteem, and experienced trauma.

Validity of the Scale and Its Subscales

The negative correlation of Social Desirability with Stockholm Syndrome and its three subscales means that one would more likely make Type II than Type I errors in diagnosing Stockholm Syndrome when using the Stockholm Syndrome scale. That is, errors would more likely be made in the direction of clients minimizing their extent of Stockholm Syndrome than in the direction of clients magnifying it. These negative correlations indicate that women perceive Stockholm Syndrome characteristics as undesirable. Such findings are consistent with others' observations (Browne, 1987; Walker, 1979) regarding victims' denial of having been abused and with the Stockholm Syndrome theory itself (which argues that abuse is denied or minimized).[7]

Support for the concurrent validity of the scale and each of its three subscales was demonstrated. As expected, the overall scale associated significantly with indicators of distress in relationships (namely, being separated, number of separations, partner hurting the women's feelings when angry, and the number of times that the partner had been so angry). Findings regarding racial differences were consistent with Bart and O'Brien's (1985) findings that Black women were more likely than White women to fight back against male rapists and to avoid rape. (See also Allard, 1991.) The overall Stockholm Syndrome scores of Asian women were nonsignificantly higher than those of Black and White women, though the nonsignificance was probably due to the small number of Asian women in the study. The higher scores of Asian women may be explained by the stronger emphasis that Eastern cultures, as compared to Western cultures, place on maintaining harmonious relationships (Singelis, 1994).

Consistent with expectation, the scale and its subscales failed to correlate with the Reasoning scale of the CTS while correlating positively with the IES, the BPD scale, the PLS, and the two violence scales of the CTS, though the correlations of Love-Dependence with BPD and Physical Violence were so low as to possibly lack meaningfulness. Consistent also with our characterizations of the subscales, Core Stockholm Syndrome correlated most strongly with the IES ($r = .82$), suggesting that it indeed does measure responses to interpersonal trauma. Psychological Damage correlated most highly with the BPD scale ($r = .48$), suggesting that many of its items are indeed assessing BPD characteristics, and Love-Dependence correlated most strongly with the PLS ($r = .62$), suggesting that this subscale assesses passionate love.

It is not clear why the scale and its factors correlated more strongly with Straus' psychological violence measure than with his measure of physical violence. Perhaps this was because the college dating sample as a group experienced low levels of physical violence. Alternatively, it may be that Stockholm Syndrome does in fact relate more strongly to psychological than to physical violence.

The composite of findings described in this section provides evidence for the notion that the overall Stockholm Syndrome scale and its three subscales measure responses associated with violence and trauma in intimate interpersonal relationships. The composite of findings thereby provides support for the concurrent and construct validity of the Stockholm Syndrome scale and its individual subscales.

Relations Between the Factors

One would expect persons utilizing strategies for coping with abuse—such as the cognitive distortions measured by Core Stockholm Syndrome—to also show psychological damage owing to that abuse. Thus, the high correlation between Core Stockholm Syndrome and Psychological Damage would be expected.

Graham (1994) views the (traumatic) bond as a cognitive distortion that is maintained only when other cognitive distortions are in place (e.g., denial of abuse). Some of the cognitive distortions emerging as helping to define the Core Stockholm Syndrome subscale were: denial and rationalization of abuse, self-blame, splitting, taking the abuser's perspective, viewing the abuser as a victim, and the belief that, with sufficient love, the abuser will stop being so angry. The correlation of Love-Dependence (the bond) with Core Stockholm Syndrome (the cognitive distortions on which a bond is built) and Psychological Damage is therefore also not surprising. Interestingly, Dutton and Painter (1993) found the variables describing their abuse syndrome to be significantly intercorrelated as well.

An alternative explanation for the high correlation between Core Stockholm Syndrome and Psychological Damage is that psychological impairment, including a possible preexisting BPD, increases the likelihood of women getting into abusive relationships. This might occur because the women lack skills needed to recognize and avoid abusive partners, and/or the nature of their psychological deficits taxes relationships so that otherwise nonabusive partners are abusive with them. It may also be that Psychological Damage—a loss of sense of self, depression, and low self-esteem—makes it more difficult for young women to extricate themselves from a relationship once it has proven to be abusive. Obviously, longitudinal research on abused women is needed to help unravel the questions of cause and effect in relation to abuse and abused women's characteristics.

Is Love a Coping Strategy?

In one way, Love-Dependence performed like a typical love scale: It correlated relatively highly with the PLS. On the other hand, the Love-Dependence subscale performed like a variable associated with trauma: It correlated positively with the ES and with the Psychological and Physical Violence scales of the CTS, though the correlation with Physical Violence was quite low.

This combination of findings regarding Love-Dependence is paradoxical. Could it be that Love-Dependence, as measured here, is a strategy for coping with violence? Might the women have (perhaps unconsciously) perceived love as their only means of either escaping or minimizing the partner's abuse, as Graham (1994) proposed? Folk wisdom tells us, "Love can tame the most savage beast" and "Love conquers all." This "wisdom" is reflected in Item 20 of the Core Stockholm Syndrome subscale: "If I give my partner enough love, he will stop getting so angry at me." Could (terror-based) love be a cognitive distortion used by victims to deny fear, to cope, and, as indicated in Item 20, to find a way to escape the threat of further abuse? Is it possible that the woman feels she cannot survive without her partner's love because, though unconsciously denied, she feels that his love of her is the only thing that keeps him from being *more* abusive, perhaps even fatally so?

Graham (1994) identified a number of psychological processes that might explain victims' using the label of "love" to account for their feelings and behaviors toward the abuser:

1. As described by Bem's (1965) "self-perception theory," people interpret their own behavior, trying to make sense of it. Applied here, the theory suggests that, having denied terror as the reason for being compliant and hypervigilant toward their abuser, and not seeing any other *external* reason for these behaviors, abuse victims make the (false) assumption that they must care about or even love the abuser. Denial of terror and rationalization of abuse are components of Core Stockholm Syndrome, a subscale with which Love-Dependence correlated. (See, for example, Items 3, 7, 8, 13, 14, 26, 27, 34, 47, and 49, but also see Item 12.)

2. As described by Festinger's (1957) "cognitive dissonance theory," when contradictory feelings exist, such as feelings of both love and fear for one's partner (see Item 12 from the Core Stockholm Syndrome subscale), an inner aversive state motivates victims to seek resolution of those contradictory feelings. In this case, victims' attributing their compliant and hypervigilant behavior toward the abuser to love for him reduces this discomfort (and simultaneously reduces their feelings of terror and provides hope, as suggested by Items 30 and 43). Allen (1991) found that many of the battered women in her study experienced their feelings of love and fear, and their partner's loving and abusive behaviors, as contradictory and confusing and sought to work on these issues while at a shelter.

3. Victims who have denied their abuse-induced feelings of terror and danger must account to themselves for their now-*unexplained* high arousal level. Schachter and Singer's (1962) "two-factor theory of emotion" states that people use *environmental cues* to help them interpret *unexplained* arousal. Consistent with this theory, and even more poignant, the "misattribution view of romantic attraction" (Kenrick & Cialdini, 1977; see also Walster, 1971) posits that strong states of arousal such as anxiety or fear are likely to be misinterpreted as indicating attraction, even sexual attraction. Empirical support has amassed for this view (see, for example, Driscoll, Davis, & Lipetz, 1972; Dutton & Aron, 1974; Follingstad et al., 1988; Kenrick & Cialdini, 1977; Lo & Sporakowski, 1989).

In sum, multiple psychological processes help explain why victims might use the label of love—a cognitive distortion—to describe their feelings toward an abuser from whom they perceive no way to escape: Doing so helps them account for their compliant, hypervigilant behavior, for their contradictory feelings toward the abuser, and for their high arousal state. There are also two other benefits. Labeling their feelings as love provides hope and opens up a possible escape route.

Limitations of the Studies

The negative correlations of the scale and its subscales with the M-C SDS— moderate to low in size—indicate that the subjects perceived the items comprising them, and thus the syndrome, as socially undesirable. It is likely that this social desirability response bias artificially deflated people's factor scores. Yea-saying and nay-saying response biases of subjects also may have confounded findings, for most items comprising the scale are positively worded for the syndrome.

Distributions of the scale and subscale scores for these nonclinical samples were positively skewed. Items tended to have low endorsement rates and women's responses indicated they "seldom" felt or did the things described in the items comprising the scale. It is not known whether the positive skew of scale and subscale scores affected the size or significance of correlations. These two characteristics (endorsement rates and distributions of scores) suggest the scale and its subscales might function better with a clinical abused than with a nonclinical population, even though the factors were derived using data from a nonclinical student sample. However, because the factor structure of the scale was determined for a "normative" sample of college women and not a sample of women in abusive dating relationships, it is not known whether the factor structure of this scale is descriptive of Stockholm Syndrome for this latter group.

Finally, the samples used in the current studies were primarily White and, presumably, entirely heterosexual. Would similar factors and correlations have been found with samples of other races and ethnicities? With samples of lesbians and gay men? With men?

Directions for Future Research

Additional research on the construct validity of Stockholm Syndrome is needed. For example, do scales measuring the precursors of Stockholm Syndrome (Graham & Rawlings, 1991) predict Stockholm Syndrome factor scores? Do women obtain higher subscale scores than men, assuming the factor structure of the scale generalizes to men?

Tests are warranted of the factor structure, reliability, and construct validity of the Stockholm Syndrome scale with women in frankly abusive dating relationships. Do the subscales, for example, discriminate between the following groups: women who drop charges against abusing partners and those who do not; women who stand up for themselves in mediation and those who do not; those who continue to miss their partners upon separating and those who do not; and women who return to their partners following a separation and those who do not? Longitudinal research on abused women is needed to help us answer both (a) questions of cause and effect in relation to abuse and abused women's characteristics and (b) questions of the roles that violence and Stockholm Syndrome may play in the genesis of BPD.

Research is needed to help resolve these compelling, unanswered questions: (a) Do victims maintain contact with and possibly even return to abusive partners because they are attached to them (Dutton & Painter, 1993)? Or, (b) does terror cause people to bond to those from whom they see no other way to escape, due perhaps to forced continued contact (Graham, 1994; Graham & Rawlings, 1991)? And, (c) is unbonding a separation process involving mastery of steps that leads to repair of self-processes damaged by both abuse and enmeshment with an abusive partner (Allen, 1991; Rawlings, Allen, Graham, & Peters, 1994)?

Finally, research is needed to address cultural differences in women's responses to intimate violence. Do these differences help protect Black women from, and place Asian women at greater risk for, Stockholm Syndrome? Do Black women respond to abuse in qualitatively different ways than do White and Asian women (cf. Allard, 1991)? How do differences in societal power of Black versus White men, and between these men and Black women and White women—as played out in the courts and in the home—impact the efficacy of Black versus White women's responses to abuse?

NOTES

[1]The nine "hostage" groups are: hostages, concentration camp prisoners, prisoners of war, civilians held in Chinese Communist prisons, cult members, abused children, incest victims, battered women, and pimp-procured prostitutes.

[2]Follingstad and colleagues (1988) also found that women experiencing ongoing violence in their relationships with their partners reported "allowing" their partners to be more controlling of them than did women who left after the first incident of physical violence. That is, the former women were more likely to "let it happen and not actively try to stop it, even though they might not like it" (p. 174). Thus, women who were more controlled by their

partners and who were suffering ongoing physical violence did not try to stop their partners' control of them. Did they fear the partner would become more violent if they tried to stop it?

[3]Other accounts are provided by Dutton and Painter's (1993) theory of traumatic bonding and by Follingstad and colleagues (1988).

[4]When the data were analyzed using common factor analysis and an oblique rotation, three additional items loaded at least .50 on *Factor 1:* "My partner is like me, a victim of others' anger," "After I have been bad to my partner, I have felt he was right to punish me," and 'Our relationship is perfect except when my partner is angry at me." Items 13, 30, 38, and 42, while loading at least .42 on Factor 1, did not make the .50 cutoff. Four additional items also loaded on *Factor 2:* "When I feel bad, I look at myself and know that I love me" (reverse coded), "'I do not let people get to know me," 'I get up in the morning looking forward to the day" (reverse coded), and "I have a very clear picture of what my needs are" (reverse coded). Although Items 16 and 45 loaded sufficiently strongly to make the cutoff for Factor 2 when a varimax rotation was performed, they did not do so with an oblique rotation, though each loaded at least .48 on Factor 2. Although the iterated principal factor solution yielded an identical *Factor 3* subscale using varimax and oblique rotations, Item I loaded only .45 on Factor 3 when a common factor analysis with an oblique rotation was performed. No items loaded at least .50 on *Factor 4.*

[5]Interestingly, BPD correlated .34 with the IES ($n = 761$, $p < .05$), consistent with the notion that BPD is produced by trauma.

[6]Because Straus' Verbal Aggression scale includes items referring to both nonverbal and verbal acts that appear designed to affect the psychology of the victim, but that stop short of actual physical violence, this scale is herein referred to as the "Psychological" Violence scale (cf. Barling, O'Leary, Jouriles, Vivian, & MacEwen, 1987; Pan, Neidig, & O'Leary, 1994).

[7]Consistent with this notion, both the IES and the BPD scales also correlated negatively with the M-C SDS ($r = -.22$ and -.34, respectively; $p < .01$).

REFERENCES

Allard, S. A. (1991). Rethinking battered woman syndrome: A Black feminist perspective. *UCLA Women's Law Journal, 1,* 191-207.

Allen, G. (1991). *Separation issues of battered women.* Unpublished master's thesis, University of Cincinnati, Cincinnati, OH.

Arias, I., & Beach, S. R. H. (1987). Validity of self-reports of marital violence. *Journal of Family Violence, 2,* 139-149.

Barling, J., O'Leary, K. D., Jouriles, E. N., Vivian, D., & MacEwen, K. E. (1987). Factor similarity of the Conflict Tactics Scales across samples, spouses, and sites: Issues and implications. *Journal of Family Violence, 2,* 37-54.

Barnard, C. P., & Hirsch, C. (1985). Borderline personality and victims of incest *Psychological Reports, 57,* 715-718.

Barry, K. (1995). *The prostitution of sexuality.* New York: NYU Press.

Bart P. B., & O'Brien, P. H. (1985). *Stopping rape: Successful survival strategies.* New York: Pergamon Press.

Bem, D. J. (1965). An experimental analysis of self-persuasion. *Journal of Experimental Social Psychology, 1,* 199-218.

Brende, J. O. (1983). A psychodynamic view of character pathology in Vietnam combat veterans. *Bulletin of the Menninger Clinic, 47,* 193-216.

Brown, L. S . (1992). A feminist critique of personality disorder. In L. S. Brown & M. Ballou (Eds.), *Personality and psychopathology* (pp. 206-228). New York: Guilford.

Browne, A. (1987). *When battered women kill.* New York: The Free Press.

Crowne, D. P., & Marlowe, D. (1960). A new scale of social desirability independent of psychopathology. *Journal of Consulting Psychology,* 24, 349-354.

Driscoll, R., Davis, K., & Lipetz, M. (1972). Parental interference and romantic love: The Romeo and Juliet effect. *Journal of Personality and Social Psychology,* 24, 1- 10.

Dutton, D. G., & Aron, A. P. (1974). Some evidence for heightened sexual attraction under conditions of high anxiety. *Journal of Personality and Social Psychology,* 30, 510-517.

Dutton, D. G., & Painter, S. (1993). Emotional attachments in abusive relationships: A test of traumatic bonding theory. *Violence and Victims,* 8, 105-120.

Dutton, D. G., & Painter, S. L. (1981). Traumatic bonding: The development of emotional attachments in battered women and other relationships of intermittent abuse. *Victimology: An International Journal,* 6, 139-155.

Festinger, L. (1957). *A theory of cognitive dissonance.* Stanford, CA: Stanford University Press.

Flynn, C. P. (1990). Sex roles and women's response to courtship violence. *Journal of Family Violence,* 5, 83-94.

Follingstad, D. R., Rutledge, L. L., Polek, D. S., & McNeill-Hawkins, K. (1988). Factors associated with patterns of dating violence toward college women. *Journal of Family Violence,* 3, 169-182.

Graham, D. L. R., & Rawlings, E. I. (1991). Bonding with abusive dating partners: Dynamics of Stockholm Syndrome. In B. Levy (Ed.), *Dating violence: Young women in danger* (pp. 119-135). Seattle, WA: Seal Press.

Graham, D. L. R., with Rawlings, E. I., & Rigsby, R. (1994). *Loving to survive: Sexual terror, men's violence, and women's lives.* New York: NYU Press.

Hacker, F. J. (1976). *Crusaders, criminals, crazies: Terror and terrorism in our time.* New York: Bantam.

Hatfield, E., & Sprecher, S. (1986). Measuring passionate love in intimate relationships. *Journal of Adolescence,* 9, 383-410.

Hendrick, C., & Hendrick, S. (1989). Research on love: Does it measure *up? Journal of Personality and Social Psychology,* 56, 784-794.

Herman, J. L. (1992). A new diagnosis. *Trauma and recovery* (pp. 115-132). New York: Basic Books.

Herman, J. L., & van der Kolk, B. A. (1987). Traumatic antecedents of borderline personality disorder. In B. A. van der Kolk (Ed.), *Psychological trauma* (pp. 111-126). Washington, DC: American Psychiatric Press.

Horowitz, M. J., Wilner, N., & Alvarez, W. (1979). Impact of event scale: A measure of subjective stress. *Psychosomatic Medicine, 41,* 209-128.

Hyler, S. E., & Rieder, R. C. (1987). *PDQ-R: Personality questionnaire.* New York: New York State Psychiatric Institute.

Hyler, S. E., Skodol, A. E., Kellman, H. D., Oldham, J. M., & Rosnick, L. (1990).

Validity of the Personality Diagnostic Questionnaire—Revised: Comparison with two structured interviews. *American Journal of Psychiatry, 147,* 1043-1048.

Kenrick, D. T., & Cialdini, R. B. (1977). Romantic attraction: Misattribution versus reinforcement explanations. *Journal of Personality and Social Psychology, 35,* 381- 391.

Koss, M. P., Gidycz, C. A., & Wisniewski, N. (1987). The scope of rape: Incidence and prevalence of sexual aggression and victimization in a national sample of higher education students. *Journal of Consulting and Clinical Psychology, 55,* 162-170.

Lindy, J. D., with Green, B. L., Grace, M. C., MacLeod, J. A., & Spitz, L. (1988). *Vietnam: A casebook.* New York: Brunner/Mazel.

Lipari, J. A. (1992). *Borderline personality characteristics and parent-child relationships: A study of Stockholm syndrome theory of borderline personality etiology in a normative sample.* Unpublished doctoral dissertation, University of Cincinnati, Cincinnati, OH.

Lo, W. A., & Sporakowski, M. J. (1989, September). The continuation of violent dating relationships among college students. *Journal of College Student Development, 30,* 432-439.

O'Keeffe, N. K., Broackopp, K., & Chew, E. (1986, November/December). Teen dating violence. *Social Work, 31,* 465-468.

Pan, H. S., Neidig, P. H., & O'Leary, K. D. (1994). Male-female and aggressor-victim differences in the factor structure of the modified conflict tactics scale. *Journal of Interpersonal Violence, 9,* 366-382.

Rawlings, E. I., Allen, G., Graham, D. L. R., & Peters, 1. (1994). Chinks in the prison wall Applying Graham's Stockholm Syndrome theory in the treatment of battered women. In L. VandeCreek (Ed.), *Innovations in clinical practice* (Vol. 13). Sarasota, FL: Professional Resource Press.

Schachter, S., & Singer, J. E. (1962). Cognitive, social and physiological components of the emotional state. *Psychological Review, 69,* 379-399.

Schumm, W. R., & Bagarozzi, D. A. (1989). The Conflict Tactics Scales. *The American Journal of Family Therapy, 17,* 165-168.

Sigelman, C. K., Berry, C. J., & Wiles, K. A. (1984). Violence in college students' dating relationships. *Journal of Applied Social Psychology, S,* 530-548.

Singelis, T. M. (1994). The measurement of independent and interdependent self- construals. *Personality and Social Psychology Bulletin, 20,* 580-591.

Straus, M. A. (1979). Measuring intrafamily conflict and violence: The conflict tactics (CT) scales. *Journal of Marriage and the Family, 41,* 75-88.

Walker, L. E. (1979). *The battered woman.* New York: Harper & Row.

Walster, E. (1971). Passionate love. In B. L. Murstein (Ed.), *Theories of attraction and love* (pp. 85-99). New York: Springer Publishing.

Westen, D., Ludolph, P., Misle, B., Ruffins, S., & Block, J. (1990). Physical and sexual abuse in adolescent girls with borderline personality disorder. *American Journal of Orthopsychiatry, 60,* 55-66.

White, J. W., & Koss, M. P. (1991). Courtship violence: Incidence in a national sample of higher education students. *Violence and Victims, 6,* 247-256.

Chapter 6

The Reliability and Factor Structure of the Index of Spouse Abuse With African-American Women

**Doris Williams Campbell,
Jacquelyn Campbell, Christine King,
Barbara Parker, and Josephine Ryan**

V iolence is recognized as a significant health problem for women of all racial, ethnic, and socioeconomic groups. Yet, few of the instruments used to measure the frequency and severity of spousal or partner abuse have been developed and tested on representative samples of diverse groups of women. Therefore, findings from many cross-cultural and race-comparative studies may be of limited empirical and clinical value.

The Index of Spouse Abuse (ISA) is a measure of spouse abuse partially validated by Hudson and McIntosh in two studies sampling undergraduate and graduate female students enrolled in the University of Hawaii. A third sample was composed of women independently evaluated as being victims of partner or spouse abuse or as being free from such abuse (Hudson & McIntosh, 1981). The mean ages of women in these samples were 22.8 years and 29.9 years. The racial and ethnic composition of the samples was not described. While the ISA has not been used in many research and clinical applications, it has recently been used in two sizable nursing research studies conducted by members of The Nursing Research Consortium on Violence and Abuse. Subjects for these studies represented racially and ethnically diverse groups. In one of these studies (McFarlane, Parker, Soeken, & Bullock, 1992) 691 women ranging in age from 13–29 were recruited from public prenatal clinics. In the other study, 920 women who ranged in age from 14–38 were recruited from postpartum units. The women in the latter study participated in a case-control study of abuse during pregnancy and were matched on ethnicity and age. Data from this study are currently being analyzed (Campbell, 1990). The purpose of this study was to investigate the reliability and validity of the ISA when used as a research instrument with a sample of African-American women.

REVIEW OF THE LITERATURE

Race, Ethnicity, and Abuse

Race, as a way of dividing up the human species, has considerably affected our ways of looking at many aspects of life. This includes violent relationships, social support, sources of stress, and health. Genetic sources of differences in health have especially become entrenched in our understanding of the epidemiology of many disorders (Crawford, 1991). Conclusions and assumptions based on the single variable of race vary from the most casual personal encounter to complex epidemiological studies. Yet arguments have been made (a) that race is a social category and (b) that consistent patterns of morbidity and types of health problems are based on social rather than genetic factors (Cooper & David, 1986).

Ethnicity, as differentiated from race, and the attitudes and beliefs comprising ethnic culture, may be acquired through membership in a specific ethnic group. However, ethnicity is also influenced by the environment and the nature of the community in which individuals live and integrate the meanings of their experiences (Clarehout, Elder, & James, 1982; Tripp-Reimer & Dougherty, 1985). There is research on violence against women which claims to study differences among women due to ethnicity, but what is actually measured are differences and similarities by race. Consequently, ethnic differences are assumed when, in fact, a demographic attribute was measured.

When studying ethnic beliefs and norms, one is, in a sense, only taking a snapshot of what is really a linear and dynamic social history. While there exists a paucity of investigations of ethnic influences on the abuse of women, some studies (Fagan, Douglas, & Hansen, 1983; Gondolf, Fisher, & McFerron, 1988; Hampton, 1987) have been conducted on the incidence of woman abuse within different ethnic groups. Ethnic membership is a contributing variable, but not necessarily a determinate variable, with regard to the formulation of this social history. Living patterns in rural versus urban environments, or in poverty versus affluence, are highly influential factors in the development of beliefs and modes of behavior (Haraway, 1988; Torres, 1991). Additionally, gender and social class have separate as well as confounding influences with ethnicity, resulting in similarities as well as differences in individual situational responses (Lutrell, 1989). There are some factors that are common to diverse groups of women who are abused that influence the way a woman responds to and interacts with the environment and others (Campbell, 1985; Dobash & Dobash, 1981; Janoff-Bulman & Frieze, 1983).

There may be little difference in the incidence of woman abuse across ethnic groups (Campbell, 1985). A woman's understanding and response to abuse, however, are influenced by ethnic cultural norms to which she and others adhere (Campbell, 1989, 1993; Landenburger, 1989). While there may be some difference in the meaning of abuse across cultural groups, women's needs (but not the responses they receive or resources available) may be similar. Different cultural or social contexts provide different opportunities for and restrictions on women.

Research on Spouse or Partner Abuse of African-American Women

The experiences of nonmajority battered women are generally omitted from the literature (Asbury, 1987). The failure to address ethnicity and abuse in the literature is typically evidenced by: (a) omitting the description of the race or ethnicity of the women studied, (b) acknowledging that only majority women were included, or (c) including nonrepresentative proportions of nonmajority groups. Because there are no national reporting statistics on wife battering and because most studies of battered women are based on small, nonrepresentative shelter or clinical samples, few researchers have studied domestic violence issues unique to African-American women (Asbury, 1987).

One of the issues in the literature on domestic violence is that differences in ethnicity have seldom been explored. The assertion is often made that there is little variation in rates of domestic violence according to race and ethnicity, yet Straus, Gelles, and Steinmetz (1980) reported that wife abuse was 400% greater among black couples than white couples, reinforcing prevailing stereotypes about black men being more violent in their heterosexual relationships than white men. This survey, like the majority of other general violence studies, failed to take into account social class or income in calculating rates; nor did the study consider that socioeconomic differences between the races rather than race itself may explain the discrepant rates.

In a reanalysis of the 1980 results, Straus and Gelles corrected their original conclusions (Hampton, Gelles, & Harrop, 1989; Straus & Gelles, 1990). They found that in spite of an apparent overall increased risk for marital violence in black couples from the 1975 Straus and Gelles national random survey, controlling for socioeconomic status (SES) resulted in a lower rate of husband to wife violence toward black women. Unfortunately, data specific to African-American couples from the 1985 survey have not yet been published, although that survey was designed to oversample minority ethnic groups to overcome the small cell sizes in those groups of the early study.

One study designed to evaluate specifically the convergence of race and class in explaining domestic violence rates was reported by Lockhart (1985). Lockhart (1985) used a survey technique to compare the differences in the rates of wife abuse among 307 African-American and European-American women of varying social classes. Lockhart was able to demonstrate that there were virtually no differences between the races. Although a higher percentage of black women reported at least one victimization event, the median rate of violent episodes experienced by middle-class white women was somewhat higher than that experienced by middle-class black women. Similarly, McFarlane and colleagues (1992) found the same rate of abuse in the year prior to and during pregnancy, in their sample of 691 poor African-American and white pregnant women. In at least two other small-comparison group, nonprobability studies of about 200 women each (Campbell, 1989; Lewis, 1987), race and ethnicity (African American and European American) were not found to differentiate abused from nonabused women. Thus, recent reports challenge earlier assumed racial and ethnic differences in rates of domestic violence. However, little attention has been directed toward verifying how effective research instruments used to measure spouse abuse capture this construct within racial and ethnic minority groups.

The current analysis was undertaken to investigate the reliability and validity of the ISA when used with African-American women. It is necessary that this kind of study be undertaken before using an instrument when one or more of the ethnic groups upon which the instruments will be used was not well represented in the original instrument development work and/or for which separate reliability and validity data are not available. It is important that empirical measures of spouse abuse are stable or reliable when used with varying populations if generalizations are to be made from the results. Yet, high reliability does not mean high validity (Nunnally, 1978). Valid measures of spouse abuse should represent this construct as accurately for nonmajority women as for majority women if such measures are to be useful in providing an understanding of this aspect of family violence in African-American women.

Measures of Spouse or Partner Abuse

A review of the literature of measures of spouse abuse revealed a dearth of instruments specifically designed to measure the phenomena of spouse or partner abuse, despite the growing clinical and research interest in this form of family violence.

The Conflict Tactics Scale (CTS) (Straus, 1979), used the most extensively in research on wife abuse and dating violence, has extensive support for most aspects of its reliability and validity (Straus & Gelles, 1990). It has been used in national random surveys with substantial numbers of African-American adults as well as in numerous other studies with ethnically diverse samples. However, there has not been separate reliability or validity information published for African Americans. In addition, the CTS does not measure sexual or emotional abuse nor does it take into account degree of injury or who initiated the physical violence versus self-defense tactics. There is also a well-documented tendency for males to underestimate their violence on the CTS (and probably on other instruments although this has not been studied), while women tend to be painfully honest (Saunders, 1988).

Several other instruments have been developed to measure various aspects of wife abuse, including the Wife Abuse Inventory (Lewis, 1987), The Severity of Violence Against Women Scales (Marshall, 1992), the Measure of Wife Abuse (Rodenberg, 1993), and the Psychological Maltreatment of Women Inventory (Tolman, 1989), but none have been used widely in published research as yet and none have psychometric data published specific to racial or ethnic groups. The proportion of African Americans in the instrument development samples of those four instruments ranged from 6% to 16.4%.

Other researchers have obtained data on the frequency of partner abuse using unstructured interviews or questionnaires or survey data from police department investigator's reports, and national crime statistics. It remains very difficult to locate adequately designed and empirically tested measures of spouse or partner abuse.

In part to address these problems, Hudson and McIntosh (1981) developed and tested another measure of spouse abuse that includes sexual and emotional abuse. The ISA has been used in several studies of wife abuse, and has the advantage of measuring sexual and emotional abuse and other aspects of coercive control, as well as physical abuse. Initial efforts by Hudson and McIntosh to validate the ISA provided strong support for its use as a valid and reliable measure of the degree of the abuse inflicted upon women by their male partners. The authors recognized that one of the shortcomings of the ISA was that a large proportion of the women in the abused group were from shelter populations. Therefore, the women in the abused group probably represented women who were severely abused (Hudson & McIntosh, 1981). The ISA is further described under the instrument section of this chapter.

METHOD

Subject Recruitment

Self-reported data were collected during 1990–1993 from 504 African-American women recruited from public prenatal clinics, postpartum units, and by newspaper advertisements and bulletin board postings in four urban locations: Detroit, MI; Springfield, MA; Baltimore, MD; and Tampa, FL. The women from Springfield,

Baltimore, and Tampa *(n* = 340) participated in studies of abuse during pregnancy. The women from Detroit participated in a longitudinal study of women's responses to battering. None of the women from any of the samples were shelter residents. However, the entire sample from Detroit *(n* = 164) was recruited on the basis of having a report of more than one incident of physical violence from an intimate partner during the past year. Each woman responded to a semi-structured interview, an abuse screen, and completed both scales of the ISA.

Instruments

Physical and emotional abuse were measured using the ISA and a semi-structured interview that also asked about abuse experienced by the women. Included on the interview were questions from the Abuse Assessment Screen (AAS) designed by the Nursing Research Consortium on Violence and Abuse (Parker & McFarlane, 1991). The current analysis presents results based only on responses of the women to the ISA.

The ISA is a 30-item scale designed to measure the severity or magnitude of physical and nonphysical abuse inflicted upon a woman by her spouse or partner. The ISA can be completed by most women in about 5 minutes. For each item in the questionnaire the woman responds on a scale from 1 (never) to 5 (very frequently). The ISA items represent varying degrees of abuse, taken into account in the weighted scoring and interpretation of the responses. Two scores are computed for each respondent: an ISA-P score that represents the severity of physical abuse and an ISA-NP score that represents the severity of nonphysical abuse. Scores on both scales range from 0 to 100.

The ISA was initially validated in three studies by Hudson and McIntosh (1981). The first study was composed of 398 graduate and undergraduate female students from the University of Hawaii who were married, residing with a male partner, or involved with a male partner in an ongoing relationship. The mean age of the women was 22.8 years, and 79.3% were single. They had completed 14.6 years of school and their average monthly income in 1981 was $1,447. Hudson and McIntosh did not report the race and ethnic makeup of the sample.

The Hawaii sample (HSAS) was used by Hudson and McIntosh (1981) to evaluate the factorial validity of the ISA and to estimate reliability. A principal component factor analysis procedure with a varimax rotation was used to confirm the two dimensions of the ISA that were designed to measure physical and nonphysical abuse. Factors with eigenvalues of 1 or higher were chosen. The Index of Marital Satisfaction (IMS) was used to assist the researchers in looking at both the convergent and discriminant validity of the items on both scales.

The second Hudson and McIntosh sample comprised 188 graduate and under-graduate students and a few faculty members at the University of Hawaii. Ethnicity was not specified. This sample was used to calibrate the ISA items in terms of perceived degrees of seriousness of the abusive behaviors.

The third sample of 107 consisted of women who had been classified by experienced therapists as being victims of partner or spouse abuse *(n = 63)* and women who were classified as being free of any clinically significant spouse or partner abuse *(n = 43)*. Women in the third sample were recruited from social agencies and protective shelters in Hawaii, Michigan, California, Arkansas, New Mexico, and Pennsylvania. Their mean age was 29.9 years, 54.7% were married, and 31.1% were separated or divorced. Only 14.2% were single. The mean level of school completed by these individuals was 13.4 years and the average monthly family income was $1,142. This sample the ISA-Validation sample (ISAV), was used to investigate the reliability of the ISA and to establish clinical cutting scores for the physical and nonphysical abuse subscales (Hudson & McIntosh, 1981).

Hudson and McIntosh (1981) found high correlations between the two subscales (ISA-P and ISA-NP) of the ISA. They suggested that since most of the women in the validation abused group were obtained from protective shelters, it was likely that they had experienced a great deal of both physical and nonphysical abuse. They were unable to demonstrate empirically the necessity for retaining both the physical abuse and nonphysical abuse scales comprising the instrument. They suggested that the nature of the sample may have represented a sampling bias generating a spuriously high correlation between the physical abuse and nonphysical abuse scales, since women who have been severely physically abused have also likely experienced considerable emotional abuse. While retaining the two subscales based on lower correlations *(r = .66)* of the two scales in a nonshelter sample, the authors of the ISA recommended cautious use of the ISA until further evidence is available on which to justify the retention on the two subscales (Hudson & McIntosh, 1981). The same sampling bias also made it difficult to justify the differential item weights used in scoring of the ISA.

The ISA has been tested against clinical interviews to assess for abuse. McFarlane and colleagues (1992) compared women identified as abused using a straightforward 5-item questionnaire, the AAS, and their scores on the ISA-P and the ISA-NP. African-American women identified as abused on the AAS had a mean score of 12.2 on the ISA-P and 20.48 on the ISA-NP compared to nonabused women's scores of 1.97 on the ISA-P and 5.78 on the ISA-NP.

There is further support for the construct validity of the ISA subscales (Campbell, 1994). One approach to construct validation is evidence of convergent validity (Polit & Hungler, 1991). Campbell (1994) used the ISA subscales as well as the Danger Assessment (DA) as measures of abuse in a sample of 381 women. Represented in the sample of a low-income clinic population were 48% African-American, 24% Hispanic, and 24% Anglo-American women. A nonethnic specific analysis revealed correlations between the DA and ISA-P of .767 and between the DA and NP of .665. These correlations are sufficiently high to suggest that the DA and ISA subscales are measures of the same construct.

RESULTS

Descriptive

Subjects. Participants in this study were 504 African-American women. They were similar on most demographic variables with the exception of age. Results are generally reported on 485 cases based on a listwise deletion of cases with missing data using the statistical package SPSS-X.

The women ranged in age from 14 to 42 years. Adult women ranged in age from 20 to 42 with a mean age of 25.5 years, $SD = 5.5$. Teens comprised one third of the sample. They ranged in age from 14 to 19 (X = 17.5, SD = 2.3) and differed significantly from adult women on only one of the two scales of the ISA. Teens scored lower than adult women on the Index of Spouse Abuse-Physical (ISA-P) (8.25 vs. 15.82, $F = 21.51, p < .001$), suggesting less severe physical abuse reported by teens. The decision to include teens in the composite sample is based on reports of the dynamics of violence in adolescent partner relationships (Koval, 1989; Makepeace, 1981). The dynamics of violence for teens are similar to those for violence in adult partner relationships relating to coercive power and control.

There were no statistically significant differences in education, income, and ISA scores across data collection sites using chi-square tests. The mean educational level for the composite sample was 12.5, SD = 2.9. Sixty-eight percent of the women qualified for the Medicaid and WIC programs within their states. The remaining women, primarily the Detroit subsample, had more moderate incomes (X = $14,478, SD = $17,200). However, the median family income for the Detroit subsample was only $7,200 per year.

ISA Scores

The clinical cutting scores recommended by Hudson and McIntosh (1981) for the Index of Spouse Abuse–Physical (ISA-P) and the Index of Spouse Abuse–Nonphysical (ISA-NP) subscales are 10 and 25 respectively. These clinical cutting scores were found to minimize the sum of false positives and false negatives. The classification error rate for the total clinical criterion sample was 9.3% (Hudson & McIntosh, 1981). Over one third of the African-American women (AAW) in our composite sample were above the cutting scores for physical abuse (ISA-P) and a similar frequency was reported for nonphysical abuse (ISA-NP) (Table 1).

The mean score for the composite sample on the ISA-P scale was 15.63 *(SD =* 21.98). Scores ranged from 0 to 100. The mean score for the composite sample on the ISA-NP was 21.86 *(SD* = 24.54) and scores ranged from 0 to 96.46. Such variability is frequently observed in studies of wife abuse (Lockhart, 1985). Several factors account for the large variability. One fourth of the women in this sample were recruited into the study on the basis of having been abused during the past year. The large variability is also likely associated with the method by which items are

**TABLE 1. Frequency, Percent, and Median Rates of Physical and
Nonphysical Abuse in Sample of African-American Women**

Variable	Frequency	Percent	Median
Physical abuse ($N = 485$)			3.62
No	299	61.6	
Yes	186	38.4	
Nonphysical abuse ($N = 473$)			11.37
No	318	67.2	
Yes	155	32.8	

Note. Variations on N reflect deletion of cases with missing data.

weighted and scored on each of the ISA subscales. Items are weighted to account for levels of intensity and severity of abuse. For these reasons, median scores are also reported for our sample as the most appropriate measure for a skewed distribution and when one is interested in finding a typical value. The results were ISA-P, Md = 3.6 (5th percentile = .000, 95th = 65.49); ISA-NP, Md = 11.36 (5th percentile = .000, 95th = 73.69). Findings of the extent to which female university students in the HSAS sample were abused by their male partners were not reported in 1981 pending replication of the study at another university.

The correlation between the ISA-P and the ISA-NP was high *(r* = .88, *p* = .001) for this sample. Hudson and McIntosh (1981) also reported a high correlation between the two subscales *(r* = .86). They attributed the high correlations to the nature of the group used to validate the ISA subscales, a shelter group. The current sample of African-American women were, however, totally a nonshelter sample. A lower correlation between the ISA-P and the ISA-NP *(r* = .66) in Hudson and McIntosh's Hawaii sample (HSAS) supported the 1981 decision not to treat the ISA as a unidimensional scale.

Reliability

Alpha coefficients on the ISA-P and the ISA-NP for the current sample were .93 and .95 respectively. For the HSAS sample the ISA-P and ISA-NP alpha coefficients were .9031 and .9123, and .9420 and .9688 for the ISAV sample (Hudson & McIntosh, 1981).

Factorial Validity

The factorial validity of the ISA was evaluated using the unweighted item scores from the sample of African-American women (AAW). A principal components factor analysis procedure with a varimax rotation was used. The factor analysis procedure replicated the approach used by Hudson and McIntosh (1981) on data from the Hawaii sample (HSAS). In the same manner, all factors with eigenvalues of 1.0 or greater were extracted in the current study. Three factors were extracted.

The rotated factor loadings obtained by Hudson and McIntosh using data from the HSAS sample can be compared with the factor loadings obtained by the current researchers on two factors: physical abuse and nonphysical abuse (Table 2). A third factor was extracted from the data on the African-American women (Table 2). Factor 1 (Nonphysical) accounted for 54.5% of total variance in ISA scores. The

TABLE 2. Factor Loadings on Dimensions of the ISA[a]

Item	Nonphysical Abuse (Factor 1)		New Factor (Factor 2)	Physical Abuse (Factor 3)	
	HSAS 1981	AAW 1993	AAW 1993	HSAS 1981	AAW 1993
ISAI	**.58**	**.72**	.38	.36	.14
ISA2	**.57**	**.59**	.49	.25	.29
ISA3	.05	**.41**	.36	**.57**	.34
ISA4	.14	.14	.40	**.77**	**.58**
ISA5	**.61**	**.55**	.33	.11	.36
ISA6	**.64**	.23	**.71**	.16	.16
ISA7	.36	.48	.23	**.71**	**.57**
ISA8	**.36**	**.72**	.07	.01	.32
ISA9	**.71**	**.67**	.20	.41	.32
ISAIO	**.78**	**.61**	.45	.24	.28
ISA11	.42	**.67**	.34	**.49**	.33
ISA12	.67	.53	**.54**	.37	.12
ISA13	.01	.22	.18	**.74**	**.75**
ISA14	**.61**	**.53**	.48	-.02	.19
ISA15	**.59**	**.72**	.31	.33	.22
ISA16	**.48**	.36	**.42**	.14	.29
ISA17	.04	.29	.10	**.77**	**.74**
ISA18	**.42**	.19	**.45**	-.04	.29
ISA19	.45	.35	**.53**	**.46**	.14
ISA20	**.48**	.16	**.73**	.04	.17
ISA21	**.61**	.32	**.59**	.25	.40
ISA22	.45	**.64**	.46	**.51**	.29
ISA23	.20	.49	.27	**.86**	**.60**
ISA24	.06	.44	.38	**.71**	**.48**
ISA25	**.63**	**.70**	.39	.53	.36
ISA26	**.62**	**.61**	.50	.33	.27
ISA27	.48	**.73**	.38	**.69**	.37
ISA28	.31	**.60**	.39	**.71**	.46
ISA29	**.56**	**.74**	.22	.49	.42
ISA30	.30	.45	.37	**.72**	**.51**

Note. N = 498 HSAS sample; N = 485 AAW sample.
[a]For each item, the highest loadings for the HSAS and AAW samples are indicated in boldface.

second factor, named "New Factor" (NF), extracted from the data on the African-American women suggests that for this sample, 6 of the 30 items considered as indicators of abuse for Hudson and McIntosh's factorial validation sample were either not perceived as indicators of either physical or nonphysical abuse by the African-American sample or perceived differently. This factor explained 4.1% of the variance in ISA scores. Factor 3 (Physical abuse) only explained 3.5% of the variance. Together, Factors 1 (Nonphysical), 2 (New Factor), and 3 (Physical) explained 62.0% of the variance in ISA scores of the African-American women. Hudson and McIntosh (1981) did not report separate proportions of variance by factor. However, they did report that the three factors extracted (IMS-Index of Marital Satisfaction; P-Physical abuse; and NP-Nonphysical abuse) were present among the 55 items that explained 55.8% of the total item variance.

A comparison of the factor loadings in the Hawaii (HSAS) sample and the African-American women (AAW) sample is presented in Table 2. The cutoff loading for factor designation was .40. For each item, the highest loadings for the Hawaii (HSAS) sample and the African-American women (AAW) sample are highlighted.

During the 1981 validation studies, Hudson and McIntosh specified a priori that items 7, 13, 17, 23, 24, and 30 were marker items for the physical abuse factor and items 1, 2, 5, 6, 8, 9, 10, 14, 15, 16, 18, 19, 20, 26, and 19 were regarded as marker items for the nonphysical abuse factor. The remaining items were assigned post hoc as measures of physical or nonphysical abuse depending upon the sizes of their loadings on the two abuse factors. Thus, the final instrument included a 12-item physical abuse scale and an 18-item nonphysical abuse scale.

Similarities and differences in scale items between the two samples (HSAS) and (AAW) are presented in Table 3. Item weights used in scoring the scales are in parentheses following each item. Low item weights indicate less severe abuse. The most severe acts of abuse show the highest item weights. The scoring formula is well described by Hudson and McIntosh (1981). Differences based on item loadings for the African-American women are highlighted.

DISCUSSION

Although poor, minority women may appear to be at greater risk, battering is neither confined to, nor explained by, poverty or race (Campbell, 1993). The data shown in Table 1 indicate that if the ISA is a valid and reliable measure of spouse or partner abuse of African-American women, that such abuse is a common occurrence in this sample of primarily poor women. However, because over one fourth of the sample in this analysis was from a study of abused women (Detroit subsample), it is important to emphasize that the high rate of women above the cutting scores does not indicate the rate of abuse in the general population of African-American women. In fact, a study of all women entering public prenatal clinics in Baltimore, MD, and

TABLE 3. Similarities and Differences in Item Indicators of Spouse Abuse in 1981 HSAS Sample and 1993 AAW Sample[a,b]

		Scale 1981 HSAS	Scale 1993 AAW
ISA1	My partner belittles me. (1)	NP	NP
ISA2	My partner demands obedience to his whims. (17)	NP	NP
ISA3	My partner becomes surly and angry if I tell him he is drinking too much. (15)	P	**NP**
ISA4	My partner makes me perform sex acts that I do not enjoy or like. (50)	P	P
ISA5	My partner becomes very upset if dinner, housework, or laundry is not done when he thinks it should be. (4)	NP	NP
ISA6	My partner is jealous and suspicious of my friends. (8)	NP	**NF**
ISA7	My partner punches me with his fists. (8)	P	P
ISA8	My partner tells me I am ugly and unattractive. (26)	NP	NP
ISA9	My partner tells me I really couldn't manage or take care of myself without him. (8)	NP	NP
ISA1O	My partner acts like I am his personal servant. (20)	NP	NP
ISA11	My partner insults or shames me in front of others. (41)	NP	NP
ISA12	My partner becomes very angry if I disagree with his point of view. (15)	NP	NP
ISA13	My partner threatens me with a weapon. (82)	P	P
ISA14	My partner is stingy in giving me enough money to run our home. (12)	NP	NP
ISA15	My partner belittles me intellectually. (20)	NP	NP
ISA16	My partner demands that I stay home to take care of the children. (14)	NP	**NF**
ISA17	My partner beats me so badly that I must seek medical help. (98)	P	P
ISA18	My partner feels that I should not work or go to school. (21)	NP	**NF**
ISA19	My partner is not a kind person. (13)	NP	**NF**
ISA20	My partner does not want me to socialize with my female friends. (18)	NP	**NF**
ISA21	My partner demands sex whether I want it or not. (52)	NP	**NF**
ISA22	My partner screams and yells at me. (38)	P	**NP**
ISA23	My partner slaps me around my face and head. (80)	P	P
ISA24	My partner becomes abusive when he drinks. (65)	P	P
ISA25	My partner orders me around. (29)	NP	NP
ISA26	My partner has no respect for my feelings. (39)	NP	NP
ISA27	My partner acts like a bully towards me. (44)	NP	**NP**
ISA28	My partner frighten me. (55)	P	**NP**
ISA29	My partner treats me like a dunce. (29)	NP	NP
ISA30	My partner acts like he would like to kill me. (80)	P	P

Note. P = physical scale (1981); NP = nonphysical scale (1981); NF = new factor—AAW sample. [a]Item weights used in scoring the scales are in parentheses after each item. [b]Differences with 1993 AAW sample are in boldface.

Houston, TX, found a rate of abuse in the year prior to pregnancy of 29% for African-American women and a rate of abuse during pregnancy of 19%. Similar prevalence rates were found for Anglo-American women in the same study.

While the current study included only one ethnic group, African-American women, ethnicity is probably only one of several variables, interacting with others (e.g., SES) which might contribute to how women define and respond to domestic violence (Asbury, 1993; Haraway, 1988; Torres, 1991). Our study did not represent diverse levels of SES among the participants, and in this respect suffers from the same limitations of other studies which tend to overrepresent poor women in samples. The women in each of our subsamples are women whose mean family incomes fall below the mean and median family incomes for blacks in each of the cities from which they were recruited (U. S. Department of Commerce, 1993).

Reliability and Subscale Correlations

The alpha reliability coefficients on the physical and nonphysical scales of the ISA with African-American women are certainly impressive. Such high reliability coefficients suggest that each of the subscales is of homogeneous items. High correlations between the two scales found in this study were also reported by Hudson and McIntosh (1981) who suggested that the women in their validation sample (primarily women in protective shelters) had likely experienced a great deal of both physical and nonphysical abuse. A similar sampling bias may be represented in our Detroit subsample since these women were recruited on the basis of having a report of more than one incident of physical violence from an intimate partner during the past year. It is likely that for this subsample, at least, the women had experienced not only physical violence, but emotional or psychological abuse as well.

Factor Validity

The most important finding of this study is that with low-income African-American women there are three factors rather than two on the ISA. Ten out of 30 items on the ISA load on different factors for the current sample, compared with loadings for the original samples of Hudson and McIntosh. Thus, the factor structure found with this sample demonstrates a different interpretation of many of the items than that found in the original instrument development work.

The factor loadings for some items with this sample are actually more logical than that found in the original factor analysis. As can be seen in Table 3, five of the items on the original physical abuse factor (e.g., #22 "My partner screams and yells at me") seem misplaced for the African-American women (others are items 3, 19, 27, 28). In contrast, all of the a priori designated physical violence items loaded highest on the same factor in the current factor analysis, along with only one item not specifically describing a physically violent act, Item #30 "My partner acts like he would like to kill me." However, this item refers to the most potentially serious behavior of all the items except for "threatening with a weapon" and is certainly consistent with that item. Thus the factor division between nonphysical and physical abuse that was revealed in this factor analysis demonstrates support for the validity of the instrument in this sample.

The differences between the "new factor" and the nonphysical factor are not as easily identified. Except for Item #19 ("My partner is not a kind person"), the new factor items seem to be behaviors of an extremely controlling and isolating nature rather than the more emotional or psychological abuse represented on the nonphysical factor (e.g., #'s 1 and 15 relating to belittling). This may reflect research that suggests different typologies of batterers (e.g., Gondolf, 1988). However, the typologies may be different in different ethnic groups. For example, #19, the seemingly misplaced item in the original factor analysis, may be due to cultural differences if it is based on the Hawaii samples. The items on the "new factor" echo some of the issues that William Oliver (1989) describes when explicating the dynamics related to black male on black female violence. As Oliver (1989) states, "when black males engage in violence against black females, it is because they have defined the situation as one in which the female's actions constitute a threat to their manhood" (p. 265). Consistent with Oliver's assertions, the "new factor" item (ISA16) "My partner demands that I stay home to take care of the children" can be thought of as part of a scenario whereby if he took care of the children it would be a threat to his manhood. Similarly, item ISA18, "My partner feels that I should not work or go to school" may be part of the same manhood issue, rather than only an issue of control. Alternatively, the "new factor items" (ISA16 and ISA19) may reflect aspects of African-American culture unrelated to family violence. For example, Asbury (1993) states that the employment of African-American women is not likely to contribute to the stress that sometimes results in violence since the women have typically been part of the paid labor force. The reality for many African-American families is that women fulfill the role of coproviders or sole providers in households where both husbands and wives (or both male and female partners) are present because of underemployment or unemployment of black males (Sudarkasa, 1993). The same economic reality may lead to the male partner's support of the woman's efforts to improve her level of education and thereby increase her employment opportunities.

Demanding sex and keeping her away from, or being suspicious or jealous of, her friends (ISA 6, ISA20, ISA21) reflect behaviors related to dominance, control, and isolation. These behaviors may also represent dynamics similar to those described by Oliver (1989), since controlling sex is certainly a manhood issue and women are often seen by black men as "trying to make them look bad in the eyes of others" (p. 265). Although the manhood issue is salient for white batterers also, it is especially an issue for black men who so often cannot assert a traditional male role of proud provider because of discrimination and disdain in this society. Thus, it makes sense that this "new factor" might emerge for an African-American sample and this would be an interesting avenue to further explore with African-American battered women. At the same time, this factor only explained 4.1% of the variance in the scores on the ISA in this population. By far, the largest proportion of the variance in scores on the ISA was the nonphysical abuse factor.

Thus, the factor structure of the ISA (Hudson & McIntosh, 1981) in this African-American sample, although substantially different from the original, is understandable and actually supportive of the use of the instrument with African-American women.

Further Validation of the ISA

In 1990, Hudson continued development and validation of instruments to measure a wider range of partner abuse. The 1990 instruments represent substantial revisions of the original ISA (Hudson, 1990a, 1990b). The revision resulted in the Partner Abuse Scales, which are essentially two separate instruments: one measuring physical abuse (Partner Abuse Scale Physical—PASPH); and one measuring nonphysical abuse (PASNP). Each scale is composed of 25 items and scores range from 0–100. The new scales were designed to be used with both heterosexual and homosexual couples who are dating or who live together as married or as unmarried couples. The new scales were partially validated by Attala, Hudson, and McSweeney (1994) and estimated cutting scores for a determination of probable abuse were reported.

CONCLUSIONS

This study demonstrates the need to critically examine and evaluate instruments developed to measure the frequency and severity of spouse or partner abuse. The instruments should be studied to investigate the extent to which they are reliable and valid measures of the concept of spouse or partner abuse when used with diverse populations who may not have been represented in the samples used for initial instrument development and validation studies.

We found the ISA to be useful as a research measure of the degree and magnitude of abuse reported by African-American women. However, the substantially different findings related to the factor structure of the ISA when used with primarily poor African-American women suggest a cautious interpretation of findings when the instrument is used with this group.

It is important that the relationship between culturally valid instrumentation and generalizability not be underestimated (Porter & Villarruel, 1993). Thus, while the findings of this study may generalize, with caution, to groups of poor African-American women, they may not generalize to other groups of African-American women of different social and economic groups.

Future studies are warranted to determine how much variance in abuse is explained by ethnicity and other relevant cultural variables while controlling for

SES across all levels of SES when using instruments designed to measure partner or spouse abuse. Also needed are studies that examine how structural stressors such as poverty, joblessness, lack of education, and living in rural versus urban environments translate into intrafamily violence, especially among African Americans and other ethnic minorities in America. When such studies are conducted, it is imperative that the measurement instruments are accurate and appropriate for use with different ethnic and cultural groups and that items are consistently interpreted within and across ethnic and cultural groups.

Instrument development, reliability, and validity issues represent challenges for researchers seeking to study diverse populations. As suggested by Porter and Villarruel (1993), continued efforts must be made to psychometrically establish the validity and reliability of instruments for populations under study. This study reflects such an effort. Only when research methodologies lead to clear conceptualizations of the experiences of abuse by African-American and other ethnic, minority women can further examination of issues unique to these groups be studied and appropriately addressed.

REFERENCES

Asbury, J. (1987). African-American women in violent relationships: An exploration of cultural differences. In R. Hampton (Ed.), *Violence in the black family: Correlates and consequences* (pp. 89-104). Lexington, MA: Lexington Books.

Asbury, J. (1993). Violence in families of color in the United States. In R. Hampton, T. Gullotta, G. Adams, E. Potter, & R. Weissberg (Eds.), *Family violence: Prevention and treatment* (pp. 159-175). Newbury Park, CA: Sage Publications.

Attala, J., Hudson, W., & McSweeney, M. (1994). A partial validation of two short-form partner abuse scales. *Women and Health, 21*(2/3), 125-138.

Campbell, D. (1993). Nursing care of African-American battered women: Afrocentric perspectives. *AWHONN'S Clinical Issues, 4*(3), 407-415.

Campbell, J. (1985). Beating of wives: A cross cultural perspective. *Victimology: An International Journal, 10*(1-4), 174-185.

Campbell, J. C. (1989). A test of two explanatory models of women's responses to battering. *Nursing Research, 38,*18-24.

Campbell, J. C. (1990). *Birthweight and abuse during pregnancy: A nursing analysis of cultural influences* (National Institutes of Health, Contract No. R01 NR02571).

Campbell, J. C. (1994). *Assessing the risk of dangerousness: Violence by sexual offenders, batterers and child abusers.* Thousand Oaks, CA: Sage Publications.

Clarehout, S., Elder, J., & James, C. (1982). Problem solving skills of rural battered women. *American Journal of Community Psychology, 10,* 605-612.

Cooper, R., & David, R. (1986). The biological concept of race and its application to public health and epidemiology. *Journal of Health Policy Law, 11*(1), 97-116.

Crawford, M. (1991). The raging bull of Berkeley. *Science, 251,* 368-371.

Dobash, R., & Dobash, R. (1981). Social science and social action: The case of wife beating. *Journal of Family Issues, 2,* 439-470.

Fagan, J. A., Douglas, K.S., & Hansen, K. Y. (1983). Violent men or violent husbands? Background factors and situational correlates. In D. Finkelhor, R. Gelles, G. Hotaling, & M. Straus (Eds.), *The dark side of families* (pp. 49-67). Beverly Hills, CA: Sage.

Gondolf, E. W. (1988). Who are those guys? Toward a behavioral typology of batterers. *Violence and Victims, 3*(3), 187-203.

Gondolf, W., Fisher, E., & McFerron, R. (1988). Racial differences among shelter residents. *Journal of Family Violence, 3*(1), 39-51.

Hampton, R. (1987). Family violence and homicide in the black community. Are they linked? In R. Hampton (Ed.), *Violence in the black family: Correlates and Consequences* (pp. 135-156). Lexington, MA: Lexington Books.

Hampton, R., Gelles, R., & Harrop, J. (1989). Is violence in black families increasing? A comparison of 1975 and 1985 national survey rates. *Journal of Marriage and the Family, 51*(14), 969-980.

Haraway, D. (1988). Situated knowledges: The science question in feminism and the privilege of partial perspective. *Feminist Studies, 14,* 575-599.

Hudson, W. W.. (1990a). *Partner abuse scale: Non-physical (PASNP).* Tempe, AZ: Walmyr Publishing Company.

Hudson, W. W. (1990b). *Partner abuse scale: Physical.* Tempe, AZ: Walmyr Publishing Company.

Hudson, W.W., & McIntosh, S. (1981). The assessment of spouse abuse: Two quantifiable dimensions. *Journal of Marriage and the Family, 43,* 873-888..

Janoff-Bulman, R., & Frieze, I. H. (1983). A theoretical perspective for understanding reactions to victimization. *Journal of Social Issues, 39*(2), 1-17.

Koval, J. E. (1989). Violence in dating relationships. *Journal of Pediatric Health Care, 3*(6), 298-304.

Landenburger, K. (1989). A process of entrapment in and recovery from an abusive relationship. *Issues in Mental Health Nursing, 10,* 209-227.

Lewis, B. Y. (1987). Psychosocial factors related to wife abuse. *Journal of Family Violence, 2,* 1-10.

Lockhart, L. L. (1985). Methodological issues in comparative racial analyses: The case of wife abuse. *Social Work Research and Abstracts, 21,* 35-41.

Lutrell, W. (1989). Working-class women's ways of knowing: Effects of gender, race, and class. *Sociology of Education, 62,* 33-46.

Makepeace, M. (1981). Courtship violence among college students. *Family Relations, 30,* 97-102.

Marshall, L. L. (1992). Development of the severity of violence against women scales. *Journal of Family Violence, 7*(2), 103-121.

McFarlane, J., Parker, B., Soeken, K., & Bullock, L. (1992). Assessing for abuse during pregnancy: Severity and frequency of injuries and associated entry into prenatal care. *JAMA, 267*(23), 3176-3178.

Nunnally, J. C. (1978). *Psychometric theory.* New York: McGraw-Hill.

Oliver, W. (1989). Sexual conquest and patterns of black-on-black violence: A structural-cultural perspective. *Violence and Victims, 4,* 257-274.

Parker, B., & McFarlane, J. (1991). Nursing assessment of the battered pregnant woman. *MCN: Journal of Maternal Child Nursing, 16,* 161-164.

Polit, D. F., & Hungler, B. P. (1991). *Nursing research: Principles and methods* (4th ed.). Philadelphia: J. B. Lippincott.

Porter, C. P., & Villarruel, A. M. (1993). Nursing research with African-American and Hispanic people: Guidelines for action. *Nursing Outlook, 41*(2), 59-67.

Rodenburg, F. A. (1993). The measure of wife abuse: Steps toward the development of a comprehensive assessment technique. *Journal of Family Violence, 8,* 202-228.

Saunders, D. G. (1988). Wife abuse, husband abuse, or mutual combat? In K. Yllo & M. Bogard (Eds.), *Feminist perspectives on wife abuse* (pp. 90-113). Beverly Hills: Sage.

Straus, M. (1979). Measuring intrafamily conflict and violence: The conflict tactics (CT) scales. *Journal of Marriage and the Family, 41,* 75-88.

Straus, M., & Gelles, R. (1990). *Physical violence in American families: Risk factors and adaptations to violence in 8,145 families.* New Brunswick: Transaction.

Straus, M., Gelles, R., & Steinmetz, S. (1980). *Behind closed doors: Violence in the American family.* Garden City, NY: Anchor/Doubleday.

Sudarkasa, N. (1993). Female-headed African-American households: Some neglected dimensions. In H. McAdoo (Ed.), *Family ethnicity: Strength in diversity* (pp. 81-89). Newbury Park, CA: Sage.

Tolman, R. M. (1989). The development of a measure of psychological maltreatment of women by their male partners. *Violence and Victims, 4,* 159-177.

Torres, S. (1991). A comparison of wife abuse between two cultures: Attitudes, nature, and extent. *Issues in Mental Health Nursing, 12*(1), 112-131.

Tripp-Reimer, T., & Dougherty, M. (1985). Cross cultural nursing research. In H. Werley & J. Fitzpatrick (Eds.), *Annual review of nursing research* (vol. 3, pp. 77-104). New York: Springer Publishing.

United States Department of Commerce. (1993). *1990 census of the population: Social and economic characteristics* (Vols. Florida, Maryland, Massachusetts, Michigan). Washington, DC: U.S. Government Printing Office.

Chapter 7

Measuring Interference With Employment and Education Reported by Women With Abusive Partners: Preliminary Data

Stephanie Riger, Courtney Ahrens, and Amy Blickenstaff

Violence by intimates may be a critical barrier to employment of a sizable proportion of welfare recipients (Allard, Albelda, Colten, & Cosenza, 1997; Nadel, 1998; Raphael, 1996). Many state welfare policies now require women to attempt to find work after a certain time period if they are to continue to receive government aid. Yet job training providers report that some men sabotage women's employment efforts by acts such as leaving visible marks of a beating on a woman just before she has a job interview or threatening her coworkers (Raphael, 1996). In recognition of the possibility of increased violence when women on welfare attempt to attain employment or education, the Family Violence Option to the 1996 federal welfare reform legislation offers states the opportunity to provide counseling and other services to women with abusive partners and temporarily to waive work and other requirements for them. The assumption underlying the Family Violence Option is that men who abuse women in other ways will also interfere with their attempts to go to work and/or to school. Yet, testing this assumption is problematic because no adequate measure exists of actions by intimates that affect women's employment or education. As many women are now reaching their two-year limit on consecutive receipt of government aid, the need for such a measure is pressing.

Some conceptualizations of violence, such as the Power and Control Wheel (Pence & Paymar, 1993) and Tolman's (1989) Psychological Maltreatment of Women Inventory include economic abuse and isolation. However, current measures of violence may not contain sufficiently specific questions about abuse related to women's attempts to become financially independent and to advance their skills and knowledge. This study assesses the validity of the Work/School Abuse Scale that measures the reported extent of partners' interference with women's employment and education.

Research on male violence against women has been hampered by the difficulty of measuring violence. Little agreement exists on how to define violence, and researchers vary in the range of behaviors they study (Crowell & Burgess, 1996). Some include only behaviors intended to harm, while others include acts that are not intended to harm but that cause damage nonetheless. Some consider only physical acts while others also include verbal and psychological abuse. The more inclusive the definition of violence, the higher the level of violence reported (Smith, 1994).

Two commonly cited sources of national data on violence against women are the National Crime Victimization Survey (reported in Bachman & Saltzman, 1995) and the National Family Violence Survey (reported in Straus, Gelles, & Steinmetz, 1980; Straus & Gelles, 1990). The National Crime Victimization Survey (NCVS) conducted by the United States government did not include specific questions about violence between intimates before 1992, at which time changes were made to increase the accuracy of reporting crimes committed by intimates or family members (Bachman & Saltzman, 1995). Behavior-specific wording replaced criminal justice terminology to make it easier for respondents to understand the meaning of questions, and items were added that included a wide spectrum of violent acts. Such methodological changes resulted in increases in reported rates of violent victimizations against women.

The Conflict Tactics Scale (CTS), developed for the National Family Violence Survey, includes measures of the use of reasoning and verbal/symbolic aggression as well as physical violence such as pushing, shoving, grabbing, kicking, biting, and so forth (Straus, 1979). Despite its frequent use, the CTS has been criticized for not specifying whether violent acts were in attack or self-defense, not taking into account the degree of injuries sustained, not sufficiently discriminating among different kinds of violence, and not recognizing the use of violence as a means of control of women (Daly, 1992; Dobash, Dobash, Wilson, & Daly, 1992; Koss, Goodman, Browne, Fitzgerald, Keita, & Russo, 1994; Kurz, 1993; cf. Straus, 1990, 1993).

In response to these criticisms, the CTS was revised to distinguish between minor and severe levels of physical force and to assess injuries incurred as a result of the abuse (Straus, Hamby, Boney-McCoy, & Sugerman, 1996). Yet, despite these revisions, several researchers continue to criticize the CTS, claiming that conceptualizing intimate violence as the use of tactics to resolve conflicts obscures the dynamic of power and control that is inherent to domestic violence (Bograd, 1988; Schechter, 1988; Yllo, 1993). These researchers argue from a feminist perspective that multiple forms of coercive control are used by abusers (and reinforced by the patriarchal nature of society) to dominate women. The Power and Control Wheel (Pence & Paymar, 1993) illustrates this spectrum of control and includes acts such as intimidation, emotional abuse, isolation, economic abuse, coercion and threats, male privilege, manipulation through the children, and minimization, denial, and blame.

In addition to the measures described above, several other instruments have also been developed to assess a wide variety of violent acts that include both physical and nonphysical maltreatment [e.g., the Index of Spouse Abuse (Hudson & McIntosh, 1981); the Wife Abuse Inventory (Lewis, 1987); the Severity of Violence Against Women Scales (Marshall, 1992); the Measure of Wife Abuse (Rodenberg, 1993); the Abusive Behavior Inventory (Shepard & Campbell, 1992); the Psychological Abuse Index (Sullivan, Tan, Basta, Rumptz, & Davidson, 1992); and the Psychological Maltreatment of Women Inventory (Tolman, 1989)]. Both the Psychological Maltreatment of Women Inventory and the Power and Control Wheel include the concept of preventing women from going to work or keeping a job, but this form of abuse is not extensively assessed.

The lack of attention to this issue may stem, in part, from the use of shelter residents as the sample in many studies of violence. Many domestic violence shelter residents may not have been employed or have attended school recently. Consequently, this issue may not be relevant to all victims. Nonetheless, when abusers do interfere with their partner's work or school participation, the consequences for the victim may be profound, serving to further isolate the victim and limit the financial resources that could enable her to leave the battering relationship. Even though these experiences may be relevant only to a subset of domestic violence victims, it is important to understand and assess such tactics.

The purpose of this study was to develop a measure of abusive acts by intimates that prevent or hinder women's employment and/or education. Previous research indicates that multiple, behaviorally specific questions yield greater disclosure by respondents (Crowell & Burgess, 1996); therefore, we attempted to be inclusive and specific in generating items for this scale. Interference with women's work and education may come not only from actions involving the use of physical force but also from acts in which force is not used but that nonetheless affect women's participation. For example, turning off an alarm clock may cause a woman to be late to work, risking her job security. Consequently, we included both items that describe the use of force and items that describe nonforceful but interfering acts. Here the Work/ School Abuse Scale (W/SAS) and its subscales are presented and its relationship to other measures of violence is examined. Since both work and school increase women's independence and financial self-sufficiency, they have been combined into one measure. However, the items are presented separately in the Appendix, so that the work or school items may be used independently.

METHOD

Participants and Procedure

Participants in this study were recruited through a larger study by the first author of domestic violence victims residing in shelters in Chicago. Although 46% of the women in the larger study ($N = 57$) reported that their abusers had forbidden them to work and 25% reported that their abusers had forbidden them to go to school, 35 respondents (61%) had been employed or gone to school during their relationship with the abuser, whether or not they had been forbidden. Of these 35 women, 15 had both been employed and gone to school during their relationship with the abuser, 18 had been employed but had not gone to school, and 2 had been in school but had not been employed. These 35 women, who had either been employed or gone to school during their relationship with the abuser, constitute the sample for the present study.

The average woman in this sample was 31 years old and had two children under 14 years of age living with her. Eleven percent were married, 83% were African American, 51% had at least a high school diploma, and 68% were receiving welfare benefits at the time of the study.

Women at 4 shelters were interviewed between February and April, 1997. However, logistical problems enabled only one woman to be interviewed from the fourth shelter. The Illinois Department of Public Aid provided demographic information on all residents of the 3 remaining shelters during February, March, and April 1997, the months during which data were collected. A comparison of the 35 women who went to school or work during their relationship with their abuser with the total population of each of these three shelters during the time of data collection indicated that participants did not differ from the general population, with two exceptions. Interviewing in Spanish was not possible; therefore the sample had fewer Latinas than representative from the one shelter that had a large Spanish-speaking population. In this same shelter, the sample was significantly more likely to be receiving welfare than the general shelter population (see Table 1). Other than these two exceptions, the sample, albeit small, represents the population of interest and therefore meets the assumption of classic test theory (Allen & Yin, 1979).

Table 1. Demographic Comparisons of Women Who Worked/Went to School With the General Shelter Population

Variable	Shelter 1			Shelter 2			Shelter 3		
	% Sample (n = 14)	% Total (n = 141)	χ²	% Sample (n = 8)	% Total (n = 179)	χ²	% Sample (n = 13)	% Total (n = 123)	χ²
Ethnicity									
African American	92.9	78.3		75.0	57.7		92.3	82.8	
Latina	0	15.2		0	24.6		0	4.9	
Caucasian	7.1	6.5	2.48	12.5	13.1	24.60***	7.7	9.0	1.22
Married	7.1	27.7	2.80	12.5	34.6	1.68	15.4	26.0	.71
Spouse was abuser	46.2	40.0	.19	60.0	39.0	.89	25.0	28.2	.05
Medicaid for self	42.9	50.4	.29	50.0	33.5	.92	46.2	58.5	.74
Medicaid for child	64.3	46.8	1.56	75.0	29.6	7.31	61.5	53.7	.29
Welfare receipt	64.3	47.5	1.43	75.0	24.6	9.94**	61.5	41.5	1.93

Table does not include the percentages of Asian, Native American, and "Other" participants, as these numbers were negligible.
*p < .05, **p < .01, ***p < .001.

There are several possible reasons for the oversampling of welfare recipients. First, the shelter staff somehow may have systematically approached more women on welfare to be participants in this study than they approached nonwelfare recipients. Second, the financial incentive of $20 to be a participant in this study may have induced more women with few resources (e.g., women on welfare) to participate. Third, women on welfare may have stayed longer at the shelter than nonwelfare recipients, giving more opportunity for them to be part of this study. Because shelter staff were unable to keep records of whom they approached, who consented, and who declined to be study participants, it is impossible to ascertain which of these possibilities accounts for the oversampling of welfare recipients in this shelter. However, because the purpose of this study was to develop a scale, not to assess a representative sample of shelter participants, the oversampling of welfare recipients is not a problem. Moreover, the long-term goal of the present study was to develop a measure that would be useful in studying the impact of welfare policies on women; therefore, overrepresentation of women on welfare may be helpful to developing a scale appropriate for this population.

MEASURES

In addition to developing a measure of work/school interference, levels of physical and psychological violence were also assessed; the psychometric properties of these measures are reported below.

Work/School Abuse Scale. A pool of 15 items was developed from discussions with domestic violence and job training providers and from a review of the literature, including anecdotal descriptions of ways that abusive men interfere with women's work and school participation. Items described both behaviors that prevent women from going to work or school and behaviors that interfere with participation once women were at work or school. Some of the items refer to the use of physical force while others do not.

Items describing work/school interference tactics were measured on a 6-point scale ranging from "never" to "more than 4 times a week." However, responses indicate that the items had low variability; that is, harassers either used a tactic frequently or did not use that tactic at all (rather than varying the frequency with which they used each tactic). Therefore, responses to the items were dichotomized. Each of the 15 items was first asked in the context of work and then in the context of school, and the parallel work/school items were combined. If an abuser had used a tactic to interfere with either a victim's work or school participation, the combined item received a "1"; if an abuser had not used the tactic to interfere with either work or school participation, the combined item received a "0." Participants in the study completed these items as well as those asking whether or not they had ever been forbidden to go to work or school, had to miss work or school as a result of the abuse, or were fired or quit as a result of the abuse.

Physical Abuse. A modified version of the physical aggression section of the Conflict Tactics Scale (CTS) (Straus, 1979) as modified by Sullivan and colleagues (1992) was used to measure physical violence by the person who caused the respondent to enter the shelter. Items assessed the frequency of actions such as being pushed, slapped, choked, beat up, and threatened or assaulted with a knife or gun. Items were measured on a 6-point scale ranging from "never" to "more than 4 times a week." Sullivan and associates (1992) reported that the modified scale had an internal consistency of .90; in our sample the internal consistency was .89 as measured by Cronbach's alpha. Even though our sample is small, it nonetheless yields a reliability estimate that is consistent with a larger sample in previous research.

Psychological Abuse Index (PAI). The Index of Psychological Abuse (Sullivan et al., 1992) assessed the frequency of psychological abuse, such as control of money and activities, verbal abuse, and threats and criticism of the respondent, friends, family, and children. Items were rated on a 6-point scale of increasing frequencies ranging from "never" to "more than 4 times a week." Sullivan and colleagues (1992) reported that the scale had an internal consistency of .97, indicating that the items reliably measure women's experiences with psychological abuse. In our sample, the IPA had an internal consistency of .89 as measured by Cronbach's alpha. Again, although our sample is small, the reliability estimate obtained is reasonably close to the one produced by a larger sample in previous research.

RESULTS

Reliability

Reliability of the Work/School Abuse Scale (W/SAS) was assessed by examining the coefficient alpha, a widely used measure of internal consistency. Analyses of the dichotomized items revealed that 3 of the 15 items had poor psychometric properties (i.e., low corrected item-total correlations, low item means, and low standard deviations). These 3 items (which asked a woman whether her abuser had sent or left something at work or school to harass her, or whether the abuser had threatened her coworkers or school friends) were omitted. The resulting 12-item scale (see Appendix) has an internal consistency of .82 (see Table 2). Coefficient alpha tends to be lower if the scale items are dichotomously coded (Allen & Yin, 1979), and if there are a small number of items in a scale (Cortina, 1993). An alpha of .82 for a 12-item scale indicates good reliability.

The sample was too small to permit factor analysis of the 12 items. However, since the items were written to represent two types of interference, the level of reliability of two subscales consisting of these two types of behaviors was examined. The Restraint Tactics subscale contained 6 items that assessed the use of

Table 2. Psychometric Properties and Frequencies for the Work/School Abuse Scale

Scale Item	Item M	Item SD	CITC[a] Scale	CITC[a] Sub-scale	Frequency (%)
Restraint Tactics					
1) Sabotage the car	.29	.46	.41	.52	29
2) Not show up for child care	.41	.48	.44	.36	41
3) Steal car keys or money	.46	.51	.45	.56	46
4) Refuse to give a ride to work/school	.51	.51	.18	.25	51
5) Physically restrain you from going to work/school	.37	.49	.64	.60	37
6) Threaten you to prevent your going to work/school	.46	.51	.57	.54	46
Interference Tactics					
1) Comes to work or school to harass you	.40	.50	.36	.42	40
2) Bothers coworkers/school friends	.20	.41	.59	.53	20
3) Lies to coworkers/school friends about you	.37	.49	.50	.56	37
4) Physically forces you to leave work/school	.26	.44	.58	.66	26
5) Lies about children's health or safety to make you leave work/school	.41	.47	.42	.39	41
6) Threatens you to make you leave work/school	.34	.48	.61	.58	34
Dropped Items					
1) Sends something to work/school to harass you	.06	.24	.14	—	6
2) Left things at work/school to harass you	.11	.32	.15	—	11
3) Threatens coworkers or school friends	.09	.28	.27	—	9

Note. N = 35. Items were scored 0= no interference; 1= interference. [a]CITC= Corrected Item-Total Correlation.

tactics that prevent the respondent from going to work or school (e.g., steal car keys or money). The Interference Tactics subscale contained 6 items that assessed the use of tactics aimed at making the respondent leave work or school (e.g., lie about children's health or safety to make you leave work/school). These subscales have internal consistencies of .73 and .77, respectively, which, for scales consisting of small numbers of items that are dichotomously coded, indicate good reliability. Table 2 presents the 12 items that constitute the W/SAS, their psychometric properties, and the percent of women who reported experiencing each tactic.

VALIDITY

The convergent validity of the W/SAS was examined by assessing the extent to which the W/SAS correlates with measures of physical abuse (modified CTS) and psychological abuse (PAI). The correlation between the W/SAS as a whole and the modified CTS physical assault subscale ($r = .43; p < .01$), and between the W/SAS and the PAI ($r = .39; p < .05$), is both positive and significant, indicating that more interference with work and school is associated with higher levels of both physical and psychological abuse. The subscales of the W/SAS are also positively correlated with the modified CTS and the PAI. Specifically, the Restraint Tactics scale is significantly related to the modified CTS physical assault subscale ($r = .37; p < .05$), indicating that the more physical abuse a woman suffers, the more the abuser tries to restrain her from going to work and/or school. The Interference Tactics scale is significantly related to both the modified CTS ($r = .38; p < .05$) and the PAI ($r = .36$, $p < .05$). Thus, the more physical and psychological abuse a woman suffered, the more the abuser also interferes with her work and/or school participation. The fact that the correlations among the W/SAS and the other measures of abuse are significant but modest (ranging from .36 to .43) indicates that these constructs are related but not identical, demonstrating the need for a separate measure of work/ school interference.

The Relationship Between Restraining and Interfering Tactics and Work or School Participation

In addition to completing items included in the W/SAS, women in the sample were asked if their abuser forbade them to work or go to school, if they missed work or school because of abuse, and if they were fired from work or dropped out of school because of the abuse. Of those 35 women who worked or went to school during their relationship with the abuser, 46% had been explicitly forbidden by their abusers to get a job. Of the 33 women who did work, 85% of them missed work because of the abuse and 52% were fired or had to quit because of the abuse. Women who were forbidden but who worked anyway did not report experiencing more Restraint or Interference Tactics than those who worked but who were not forbidden (see Table 3). However, women who reported missing work as a result of their partners' abuse experienced significantly more interference with work activities than those who did not miss work because of abuse. Specifically, women who missed work because of abuse reported significantly higher scores on the Interference scale than those women who did not miss work. Women who were fired or quit as a result of abuse reported significantly higher scores on the Restraint scale and the total W/SAS than those women who did not stop working.

School participation is also related to the W/SAS and its subscales. Of the 35 women who had gone to work or school during their relationship with the abuser, 31% were explicitly forbidden to attend school by the abuser. Of the 17 women who did go to school, 53% reported that they missed school and 35% reported having dropped out or were kicked out of school because of abuse. Women who were forbidden, but who went anyway, and women who missed school because of abuse did not report higher scores on the Restraint or Interference Tactics scales (see Table 4). However, women who reported leaving school because of abuse also reported experiencing significantly higher scores on both the Restraint and Interference Tactics scales and the total W/SAS.

DISCUSSION

These findings indicate that the W/SAS is a reliable and valid measure of interference with women's work and/or school participation. The scale has the advantage of asking explicitly about behaviors intended to interfere with women's daily activities that have not specifically been included in most other measures. The W/SAS may be used as a measure of the impact of welfare reform on women whose changed welfare status prompts them to attempt to work or go to school as well as to give a more complete picture of the ways that violence affects women's lives.

There was not a large enough sample to conduct factor analyses on the items. Therefore, the two subscales, Restraint and Interference, require confirmation in future studies. Until then, having the subscales might be useful for descriptive purposes or for conceptualizing the overall constructs. The two subscales of the W/SAS may be related differentially to work and school participation, although the small size of this sample makes these findings inconclusive. It appears that the use of tactics that interfere with women while they are at work is related to their missing work, while the use of tactics that make it difficult for them to get to work is related to being fired or quitting because of abuse. With respect to school, both types of tactics restrict women from getting to school, and those involving interference with women while they are at school are related to their leaving school.

Although the W/SAS appears to be useful, a cautionary note is in order. The small sample size limits the confidence in these findings. Due to the pressing need, given welfare reform, for a measure of abusive interference with women's work and school participation, however, this scale is put forth as a timely first step. Future studies will need to replicate these findings with a

Table 3. Relationship Between Restraint, Interference, the Total W/SAS, and Work Participation

Variable	Restraint Sub-Scale			Interference Sub-Scale			Total W/SAS Scale		
	M	SD	t	M	SD	t	M	SD	t
Forbid to go to work									
Yes (n = 16)	.48	.30		.44	.34		.46	.28	
No (n = 18)	.37	.33	.99	.23	.28	2.03	.30	.26	1.76
Miss work because of abuse									
Yes (n = 28)	.45	.31		.39	.32		.42	.28	
No (n = 5)	.37	.40	.50	.07	.15	2.22*	.22	.19	1.55
Fired from/quit work because of abuse									
Yes (n = 17)	.56	.30		.46	.36		.49	.27	
No (n = 16)	.30	.29	2.46*	.25	.25	1.65	.28	.24	2.44*

Note. Responses to Work and School Interference Scale were dichotomized (0= no interference; 1= interference). *N*s vary due to missing data. *$p < .05$. **$p < .01$.

Table 4. Relationship Between School Restraint, School Interference, the Total W/SAS, and School Participation

Variable	Restraint Sub-Scale			Interference Sub-Scale			Total W/SAS Scale		
	M	SD	t	M	SD	t	M	SD	t
Forbid to go to school									
Yes (n = 11)	.51	.35		.45	.40		.48	.35	
No (n = 24)	.37	.31	1.24	.26	.26	1.65	.32	.23	1.67
Miss school because of abuse									
Yes (n = 9)	.43	.33		.47	.34		.45	.32	
No (n = 7)	.29	.37	.85	.17	.24	2.01*	.23	.28	1.49
Dropped/kicked out of school because of abuse									
Yes (n = 6)	.62	.32		.57	.35		.59	.33	
No (n = 10)	.22	.26	2.76*	.20	.23	2.52*	.21	.20	2.94*

Note. Responses to Work and School Interference Scale were dichotomized (0= no interference; 1= interference). *N*s vary due to missing data. *$p < .05$. **$p < .01$.

larger sample to confirm the reliability and validity of this scale and its subscales. Nevertheless, the validity of this study is supported by several aspects of the results: a) the sample, although small, is representative of the population from which it is drawn; b) the estimates of reliability for the existing measures of physical and psychological abuse are similar to those found in larger samples; and c) the reliability estimates are good, especially for scales consisting of small numbers of items that are dichotomously coded. Finally, the modest (but significant) correlations between the W/SAS and the existing measures of physical and psychological abuse indicate that the W/SAS is measuring a related but different construct.

In addition to larger samples, future studies should include women from diverse settings. This sample was drawn exclusively from residents of inner-city domestic violence shelters and therefore probably represented women who were severely abused and who had few resources. It is possible that women who suffer abuse but who do not go to domestic violence shelters experience interference with work and education in ways that differ from this sample. Furthermore, the majority of women in this sample were African American. The factor structure underlying the W/SAS may differ for varying ethnic groups of women (see, e.g., Campbell, Campbell, King, & Parker, 1994), and forms of interference not included in this scale may occur to women of other ethnic or socioeconomic backgrounds.

The Family Violence Option to the federal welfare reform legislation assumes that men who are abusive to their female partners in other ways will also interfere with women's attempts to go to work and/or school. Support for this assumption comes from the significant correlations in this study between work and school interference and both physical and psychological abuse. If women with abusive partners try to go to school or get a job, they may experience high levels of interference by their partners. Thus, victims of abuse who are welfare recipients may be caught in a double bind. They are being urged to move from welfare to work, but their attempts to do so may be thwarted by their abusive partners.

Researchers have previously identified the tendency of abusive partners to discourage women from maintaining relationships with friends and family and to isolate them from outside contacts (Browne, 1987). Male violence often occurs when women attempt to leave a relationship or in other ways to assert their independence (Dobash & Dobash, 1984; Ellis, 1992; Harlow, 1991; Mahoney, 1991). Getting a job or going to school may be seen by abusers as precursors to women's leaving. The self-esteem that attends accomplishment, the new social contacts that women make, and the income they receive from work or job training all may increase women's independence and self-assertion, consequently threatening men's authority and control. Hence, attempts to become employed or to further their education may subject women to increased violence by men who abuse their female partners. The W/SAS provides a means of identifying the scope and frequency of this violence, enabling us to further understand the role of violence in women's lives.

REFERENCES

Allen, M. J. & Yin, W. M. (1979). *Introduction to measurement.* Monterey, CA: Brooks/Cole.

Allard, M. A., Albelda, R., Colten, M. E., & Cosenza, C. (1997). *In harm's way? Domestic violence, AFDC receipt and welfare reform in Massachusetts.* Boston, MA: Center for Social Policy Research, University of Massachusetts, Boston.

Bachman, R. & Saltzman, L. E. (1995, August). *Violence against women: Estimates from the redesigned survey.* NCJ-154348. Washington, DC: Bureau of Justice Statistics, U.S. Department of Justice.

Bograd, M. (1988). Feminist perspectives on wife abuse: An introduction. In K. Yllo & M. Bograd (Eds.), *Feminist perspectives on wife abuse* (pp. 11-26). Newbury Park, CA: Sage.

Browne, A. (1987). *When battered women kill.* New York: Macmillan/Free Press.

Campbell, D. W., Campbell, J., King, C., & Parker, B. (1994). The reliability and factor structure of the Index of Spouse Abuse with African-American women. *Violence and Victims, 9,* 259-274.

Cortina, J. M. (1993). What is coefficient alpha? An examination of theory and applications. *Journal of Applied Psychology, 78,* 98-104.

Crowell, N. A. & Burgess, A. W. (1996). *Understanding violence against women.* Washington, DC: National Academy Press.

Dobash, R. E. & Dobash, R. P. (1984). The nature and antecedents of violent events. *British Journal of Criminology, 24,* 269-288.

Dobash, R. P., Dobash, R. E., Wilson, M., & Daly, M. (1992). The myth of sexual symmetry in marital violence. *Social Problems, 39,* 71-91.

Ellis, D. (1992). Woman abuse among separated and divorced women: The relevance of social support. In E. C. Viana (Ed.), *Intimate violence: Interdisciplinary perspectives* (pp. 177-189). Washington, DC: Hemisphere.

Harlow, C. W. (1991). *Female victims of violent crime.* Rockville, MD: U.S. Department of Justice.

Hudson, W. W. & McIntosh, S. (1981). The assessment of spouse abuse: Two quantifiable dimensions. *Journal of Marriage and the Family, 43,* 873-888.

Koss, M. P., Goodman, L. A., Browne, A., Fitzgerald, L. F., Keita, G. P., & Russo, N. F. (1994). *Male violence against women at home, at work, and in the community.* Washington, DC: American Psychological Association.

Kurz, D. (1993). Physical assaults by husbands: A major social problem. In R. J. Gelles & D. R. Loseke (Eds.), *Current controversies on family violence* (pp. 88-103). Newbury Park, CA: Sage.

Lewis, B. Y. (1987). Psychosocial factors related to wife abuse. *Journal of Family Violence, 2,* 1-10.

Mahoney, M. R. (1991). Legal images of battered women: Redefining the issue of separation. *Michigan Law Review, 1,* 43-49.

Marshall, L. L. (1992). Development of the severity of violence against women scales. *Journal of Family Violence, 7,* 103-121.

Nadel, M. V. (1998). Domestic violence: Prevalence and implications for employment among welfare recipients. Washington, DC: U.S. General Accounting
   Office, HEHS-99-12.
Pence, E. & Paymar, M. (1993). *Education groups for men who batter: The Duluth
   model.* New York, NY: Springer Publishing.
Raphael, J. (1996). Domestic violence and welfare receipt: Toward a new feminist
   theory of welfare dependency. *Harvard Women's Law Journal, 19,* 201-227.
Rodenberg, F. A. (1993). The measure of wife abuse: Steps toward the development of
   a comprehensive assessment technique. *Journal of Family Violence, 8,* 202-228.
Schecter, S. (1988). Building bridges between activists, professionals, and researchers. In K. Yllo & M. Bograd (Eds.), *Feminist perspectives on wife abuse*
   (pp. 299-312). Newbury Park, CA: Sage.
Shepard, M. F. & Campbell, J. A. (1992). The abusive behavior inventory: A
   measure of psychological and physical abuse. *Journal of Interpersonal Violence, 7,* 291-305.
Smith, M. D. (1994). Enhancing the quality of survey data on violence against
   women: A feminist approach. *Gender and Society, 8,* 109-127.
Straus, M. A. (1979). Measuring intrafamily conflict and violence: The Conflict
   Tactics (CT) Scales. *Journal of Marriage and the Family,* 75-88.
Straus, M. A. (1990). The Conflict Tactics Scale and its critics: An evaluation and
   new data on validity and reliability. In M. A. Straus & R. J. Gelles (Eds.),
   *Physical violence in American families: Risk factors and adaptions to violence
   in 8,145 families* (pp. 49-73). New Brunswick, NJ: Transaction Publishers.
Straus, M. A. (1993). Physical assaults by wives: A major social problem. In R. J.
   Gelles & D. R. Loseke (Eds.), *Current controversies on family violence* (pp. 67-
   87). Newbury Park, CA: Sage.
Straus, M. A. & Gelles, R. J. (1990). How violent are American families? Estimates
   from the National Family Violence Resurvey and other studies. In M. A. Straus
   & R. J. Gelles (Eds.), *Physical violence in American families: Risk factors and
   adaptations to violence in 8,145 families* (pp. 95-112). New Brunswick, NJ:
   Transaction Publishers.
Straus, M. A., Gelles, R. J., & Steinmetz, S. (1980). *Behind closed doors: Violence
   in the American Family.* Garden City, NY: Anchor Press.
Straus, M. A., Hamby, S. L., Boney-McCoy, S. & Sugerman, D. B. (1996). The
   revised Conflict Tactics Scale (CTS2): Development and preliminary psychometric data. *Journal of Family Issues, 17,* 283-316.
Sullivan, C. M., Tan, C., Basta, J., Rumptz, M., & Davidson, W. S. (1992). An
   advocacy intervention program for women with abusive partners: Initial
   evaluation. *American Journal of Community Psychology, 20,* 309-332.
Tolman, R. M. (1989). The development of a measure of psychological maltreatment of women by their male partners. *Violence and Victims, 4,* 159-177.
Yllo, K. (1993). Through a feminist lens: Gender, power, and violence. In R. J.
   Gelles & D. R. Loseke (Eds.), *Current controversies on family violence* (pp. 47-
   60). Newbury Park, CA: Sage.

APPENDIX

Work/School Abuse Scale Form

The following questions are about things that _____ (ABUSER'S NAME) may have done to bother you at work or to keep you from going to work. During your relationship with _____, did he ever....

1. Come to your work to harass you?	YES	NO	N/A
2. Bother your coworkers?	YES	NO	N/A
3. Lie to your coworkers about you?	YES	NO	N/A
4. Sabotage the car so you couldn't go to work?	YES	NO	N/A
5. Not show up for child care so you couldn't go to work?	YES	NO	N/A
6. Steal your keys or money so you couldn't go to work?	YES	NO	N/A
7. Refuse to give you a ride to work?	YES	NO	N/A
8. Physically restrain you from going to work?	YES	NO	N/A
9. Threaten you to prevent your going to work?	YES	NO	N/A
10. Physically force you to leave work?	YES	NO	N/A
11. Lie about your children's health or safety to make you leave work?	YES	NO	N/A
12. Threaten you to make you leave work?	YES	NO	N/A

The following questions are about things that _____(ABUSER'S NAME) may have done to bother you at school or to keep you from going to school. During your relationship with _____, did he ever....

1. Come to school to harass you?	YES	NO	N/A
2. Bother your school friends or teachers?	YES	NO	N/A
3. Lie to your friends/teachers about you?	YES	NO	N/A
4. Sabotage the car so you couldn't go to school?	YES	NO	N/A
5. Not show up for child care so you couldn't go to school?	YES	NO	N/A
6. Steal your keys or money so you couldn't go to school?	YES	NO	N/A
7. Refuse to give you a ride to school?	YES	NO	N/A
8. Physically restrain you from going to school?	YES	NO	N/A
9. Threaten you to prevent your going to school?	YES	NO	N/A
10. Physically force you to leave school?	YES	NO	N/A
11. Lie about your children's health or safety to make you leave school?	YES	NO	N/A
12. Threaten you to make you leave school?	YES	NO	N/A

Part II

Interrelationships and Outcomes

Chapter 8

Psychological Abuse: Implications for Adjustment and Commitment to Leave Violent Partners

Ileana Arias and Karen T. Pape

P sychological abuse, frequently defined as, "verbal and nonverbal acts which symbolically hurt the other, or the use of threats to hurt the other..." (Straus, 1979, p. 77), has been shown to covary significantly with physical abuse among married couples (Follingstad, Rutledge, Berg, Hause, & Polek, 1990), dating high-school students (Molidor, 1995), and pregnant teenage and adult women (Parker, McFarlane, Soeken, Torres, & Campbell, 1993). Contrary to expectations, women have been shown to object, fear, and resent psychological abuse and its effects more than those of physical abuse (Follingstad et al., 1990; Herbert, Silver, & Ellard, 1991; O'Leary & Curley, 1986; Walker, 1984). It is surprising, therefore, that researchers have focused little attention on the occurrence and impact of psychological abuse on women's physical and mental health. Lack of empirical interest may in part be a function of the need to respond to the severe consequences of physical battering and the expectation that psychological abuse will have fewer, less severe, and more transient consequences than physical abuse. Additionally, as Vitanza, Vogel, and Marshall (1995) suggested, difficulties in operationalizing and measuring psychological abuse may have impeded progress. Notwithstanding, there has been some empirical attention devoted recently to the impact of psychological abuse on women's physical and mental health.

Aguilar and Nightingale (1994) employed a sample of 48 battered and 48 nonbattered women to examine the impact of physical abuse on women's self-esteem. While battered women were characterized by significantly lower levels of self-esteem relative to nonbattered women, psychological abuse was the only significant predictor of low self-esteem within the battered subsample. In a sample of 234 women with a history of battering, Follingstad and her colleagues (1990) found that only three of the participants had never experienced any form of psychological abuse. Seventy-two percent of the women in this sample reported that they experienced psychological abuse more negatively than physical abuse. Women who experienced psychological abuse more negatively, relative to those who experienced physical abuse more negatively, reported more fear of the partner, shame, loss of self-esteem, depression, and anxiety. Interestingly, there were no differences between women who experienced psychological abuse more negatively and those who experienced physical abuse more negatively on severity or frequency of the physical abuse they endured.

More recently, Marshall (1996) examined the physical and psychological correlates of psychological abuse among a sample of 578 women who volunteered their participation for a study of women in "bad or stressful long term relationships with a man" (p. 383). Only 13% of Marshall's sample had never been physically assaulted by the partner while 3% had never experienced an incident of psychological abuse. Higher frequencies of psychological abuse were related to higher frequencies of serious or chronic illness and visits to a physician; more frequent use of psychotherapeutic services and psychotropic medication; lower levels of relationship satisfaction and more frequent attempts to leave the partner; and lower levels of perceived power and control.

In a community sample consisting of 232 married women, Arias, Street, and Brody (1996) found that psychological abuse was a significant predictor of depressive symptomatology and problem drinking. The effects of psychological abuse on problem drinking continued to be significant even after controlling for depression. In the aforementioned sample, Arias and Street (1996) found that the negative effects of women's psychological abuse extended to their children: psychological abuse was a significant predictor of emotionally neglectful and maltreating parenting that, in turn, predicted both boys' and girls' depression and low self-esteem.

The studies reviewed suggest that psychological abuse has a negative impact on women's physical and psychological health. However, these studies did not control for the effects of physical abuse when examining those of psychological abuse. Because both forms of abuse frequently co-occur, it is difficult to obtain sizable samples of women who are only psychologically abused or only physically abused in order to examine unique effects. Statistical control is an available alternative. There appears to be only one study that attempted to statistically control for the effects of physical abuse in determining the psychological impact of psychological abuse. Kahn, Welch, and Zillmer (1993) administered the MMPI-2 to 31 battered women residing in a shelter and instructed them to indicate whether or not they had been subjected to each of nine psychologically abusive partner behaviors such as criticisms, threats, isolation, and intimidation, and nine physically abusive behaviors such as pushing, punching, hairpulling, and use of weapons. While 68% of participants scored high on the *PS* and *PK* supplementary scales (posttraumatic stress disorder scales), experience of psychological abuse only emerged as a unique predictor of the average clinical T-score when both types of abuse were included as predictors in the regression equations.

The results of investigations completed to date suggest that it is important to examine the impact of psychological abuse on women's psychological adjustment. Psychological abuse has been associated with negative psychological sequelae and ineffective coping (Arias et al., 1996). However, it is important to control for the potential confounding effects of physical abuse. In the current investigation, we were interested in the extent to which psychological abuse was related to women's psychological adjustment above and beyond the effects of their physical abuse. To the extent that terminating abusive relationships is desirable, it is also important to specify variables that facilitate or hamper battered women's attempts to leave their abusers. Because women have been shown to be more likely to leave their abusive partners as a function of abuse severity and increases in abuse frequency and severity (Herbert, Silver, & Ellard, 1991; Marshall, 1996; Strube, 1988), we were interested in the impact of psychological abuse on women's intentions to terminate their abusive relationships, again, controlling for the potential confounding effects of physical abuse. Further, we were interested in examining conditions under which severity of psychological abuse would and would not motivate women to intend to terminate their relationships. Existing literature suggests that the presence of PTSD symptomatology may be such a factor.

Walker (1984) suggested that the psychological symptoms frequently experienced by battered women overlap greatly with symptoms comprising diagnostic criteria for posttraumatic stress disorder (PTSD; APA, 1994). Assessment of PTSD among battered women indicates that, indeed, PTSD is prevalent among battered women with prevalence estimates ranging from a low of 33% (Astin, Lawrence, & Foy, 1993; Cascardi, O'Leary, Lawrence, & Schlee, 1995) to a high of 84% (Kemp, Rawlings, & Green, 1991). Variability in prevalence estimates appears to be a function of differences across studies in the method of diagnostic assessment, the population sampled, and the length of time since the traumatic event, i.e., the violent episode(s). Higher rates are more likely to result from self-report assessments among shelter women conducted immediately, e.g., 1–2 days, after a violent event. The high prevalence of PTSD among battered women merits attention since the disorder may interfere with a woman's functioning after she leaves her abusive partner and attempts to live on her own. Additionally, PTSD symptomatology may be stressful enough to interfere with women's attempts to escape abusive relationships.

PTSD has been shown to be more likely to develop among victims who engage in dissociative strategies, such as distraction, to cope during the trauma and after (Ronfeldt, Bernat, Arias, & Calhoun, 1996). Perceptions of control over stressful events and the use of problem-focused coping strategies, such as developing a plan of action, relative to the use of emotion-focused coping, such as fantasizing about good outcomes, have been shown to be more effective in reducing distress (Lazarus & Folkman, 1984). Specific to battering, Herbert, Silver, and Ellard (1991) found that battered women who remained with their abusers were more likely to employ emotion-focused strategies to cope with their abuse than women who terminated their abusive relationships. Thus, it seems reasonable to expect that women who engage in ineffective, emotion-focused coping and feel powerless or helpless may be more likely to develop PTSD symptomatology in response to abuse.

This investigation then was designed to test the following hypotheses:

1. physical and psychological abuse will be positively related;
2. psychological abuse will be a significant predictor of battered women's psychological, i.e., PTSD, symptomatology and their intentions to leave the abusive partner even after controlling for the effects of physical abuse;
3. the relationship between psychological abuse and intentions to leave the abusive relationship will be moderated by PTSD symptomatology such that the relationship will be stronger among women who do not suffer from high levels of PTSD symptomatology than among those who do; and
4. perceptions of control over the violence and type of coping strategies used in response to physical abuse will moderate the relationship between psychological abuse and PTSD symptomatology such that the relationship will be stronger for women who do not perceive themselves to be in control over their partners' violence and for women who engage in emotion-focused coping.

METHOD

Participants

Sixty-eight women currently residing in battered women's shelters in Atlanta, Georgia, and surrounding counties participated in this project. All of the women were either married for at least 1 year (61%) or had cohabited with their current partners for at least 1 year (39%). Women on average were 36 years old and had

12.60 years of education. Forty-eight percent were White American, 43% African American, 3% Latino American, and 6% Native American. Fifteen percent of the women identified themselves as Protestant, 13% Catholic, and 72% indicated "other" religious affiliations.[1] Fifty-six percent of the women were employed outside the home earning an average personal annual income of $22,000, and all had children living at home.

All assessments were conducted within 2 weeks of each woman's arrival at the shelters. Each woman completed the assessment independently, in private, and anonymously. Women were paid $10.00 each for their participation.

Measures

Conflict Tactics Scale-Form R (CTS-R). The CTS-R (Straus, 1990) is a 19-item self-report measure designed to assess the ways in which family members and intimately related partners resolve conflict. It is composed of three subscales: (1) reasoning, (2) verbal aggression, and (3) violence. Behaviors ranging from "discussed the issue calmly" to "did or said something to spite the other one" to "used a knife or gun" are assessed, employing seven response categories indicating the frequency of behavior: 1 = never, 2 = once, 3 = twice, 4 = 3–5 times, 5 = 6–10 times, 6 = 11–20 times, and 7 = more than 20 times. Participants indicated the frequency at which their partners had engaged in each of the 19 behaviors of the CTS-R during the preceding year. Scores for each of the subscales were calculated by weighting each item (i.e., multiplying the response category code [1 through 7] by the number of the item [1 through 19]), and summing the weighted items comprising each of the subscales. Total physical abuse scores could range between 135 (no violence during the preceding year) and 945 (all forms of violence occurring more than 20 times each during the preceding year). The CTS-R has been shown to be a reliable and valid measure (Straus, 1990).

Psychological Maltreatment of Women Inventory (PMWI; Tolman, 1989). The PMWI is a 58-item self-report questionnaire used to evaluate the psychological maltreatment of women. The items reflect an individual's attempt to isolate, dominate, humiliate, and threaten his/her partner and comprise two separate but related subscales: dominance/isolation (e.g., "My partner monitored my time and made me account for where I was;" "My partner tried to keep me from seeing or talking to my family") and emotional/verbal abuse (e.g., "My partner tried to make me feel like I was crazy;" "My partner insulted or shamed me in front of others"). Participants were asked to indicate the frequency at which their partners engaged in each psychologically abusive behavior during the preceding year on a scale ranging from 1 (never) to 5 (very frequently). Total PMWI scores range from 58 (no psychological abuse) to 290 (all forms of psychological abuse occurring fre-quently). Victims' reports of psychological abuse on the PMWI have been found to be characterized by high internal consistency (Dutton & Hemphill, 1992; Tolman, 1989) and free of socially desirable responding effects (Dutton & Hemphill, 1992).

Ways of Coping Checklist-Revised (WCCL-R). The WCCL-R (Folkman & Lazarus, 1985; Forsythe & Compas, 1987) is a 66-item self-report measure that assesses a range of coping strategies, including both problem-focused (e.g., "I made a plan of action and followed it;" "I changed something so things would turn out all right") and emotion-focused strategies ("I had fantasies or wishes about how things might turn out;" "I rediscovered [focused on] what is important in life"), employed to manage the internal and external demands of stressful encounters. Factor analyses conducted on a sample of college undergraduates (Folkman & Lazarus, 1985) have resulted in eight scales: one problem-focused scale, six emotion-focused scales, and one mixed scale containing both problem- and emotion-focused items. The problem-focused scale consisting of 11 items and a composite emotion-focused scale consisting of the 24 items of the six emotion-focused scales have been shown to be reliable and were employed in this investigation.

Participants were asked to indicate the extent to which they employed each strategy to cope with their partners' most recent violent episode on a 4-point Likert scale ranging from 1 (does not apply and/or is not used) to 4 (used a great deal). Scores were calculated separately for the problem- and emotion-focused coping scales by summing the ratings for the items pertaining to each scale (Forsythe & Compas, 1987). Thus, scores for problem-focused coping could range from 11 to 44, while scores for emotion-focused coping could range from 24 to 96. As problem- and emotion-focused coping are believed to be interdependent (Folkman & Lazarus, 1980, 1985), combinations of problem- and emotion-focused coping reflect differences in coping patterns, and the ratio of problem-focused to emotion-focused coping has been found to be more sensitive to interaction between cognitive appraisals and coping (Forsythe & Compas, 1987). Accordingly, the ratio of problem- to emotion-focused coping was employed. Resulting ratios could range from 44/24 or 1.83, reflecting exclusive use of problem-focused coping, to 11/96 or .11, reflecting an exclusive use of emotion-focused coping. Equal use of both types of coping strategies would be reflected by a ratio of approximately .47.

Symptom Checklist-90-Revised (SCL-90-R). The SCL-90-R (Derogatis, 1977) is a 90-item checklist assessing psychological symptomatology. Specifically, respondents are asked to indicate how much personal discomfort each symptom on the scale has caused. The SCL-90-R is a widely used instrument consisting of nine symptom dimensions: somatization, obsessive-compulsive, interpersonal sensitivity, depression, anxiety, hostility, phobic anxiety, paranoid ideation, and psychoticism. Participants were instructed to indicate how much distress each item on the SCL-90-R had caused during the preceding year on a 5-point scale ranging from 0 (not at all) to 4 (extremely). Saunders, Arata, and Kilpatrick (1990) developed a 28-item scale within the SCL-90-R that successfully discriminated between crime-related posttraumatic stress disorder (PTSD) positive and negative women. Items comprising the PTSD subscale include SCL-90-R items such as "suddenly scared for no reason," "thoughts and images of a frightening nature," "feelings of hopelessness about the future," and "your mind going blank." PTSD subscale scores are calculated by adding a participant's responses across the 28 items and dividing the total by 28, resulting in a mean item score. The mean item score for the subscale can range from 0 to 4, and a cutoff score of .89 correctly classified 89.3% of the respondents in Saunders and colleagues' study. In conjunction with a history of victimization, this cutoff score indicates the high probability that the individual will meet criteria for PTSD. Since it is recommended that diagnosis of PTSD be made on the basis of structured diagnostic interviews, we employed this SCL-90-R subscale as a continuous measure of PTSD symptomatology and not the presence or absence of the disorder *per se*.

Procedure

Participants were informed that they would be participating in a study examining the ways that women appraise relationship conflict and the various ways that couples resolve conflictual issues. All participants completed an informed consent form. Each participant was asked to complete a packet of questionnaires that included demographic information, the CTS-R, the PMWI, and the SCL-90-R. Participants then were asked to briefly describe in writing the most recent violent event in which they were the recipient of their partners' physical aggression. They were instructed to rate the extent to which they believed they had control over the violence they described on a scale from 1 (no control) to 7 (complete control) and then to indicate the likelihood that they would end the relationship on a 7-point scale, ranging from 1 ("I will never end this relationship") to 7 ("I am 100% sure that I will end this relationship").

RESULTS

Table 1 presents the means and standard deviations for the variables examined in this investigation. The women in our sample on average were characterized by fairly high levels of physical abuse and very high levels of psychological abuse. Eighty-four percent of the women reported being survivors of severe violence such as being beaten, choked, and threatened or actually assaulted with weapons. The average psychological victimization score was 202 out of a possible score of 290, suggesting that participants in this investigation survived frequent exposure to abusive behaviors assessed by the PMWI. Likewise, participants were characterized by fairly high levels of PTSD symptomatology. Indeed, 60 participants (88%) had scores of .89 or greater, the cutoff for suspected PTSD clinical criteria. Participants on average employed a moderate number of coping strategies in response to partner violence and were equally likely to rely upon emotion- and problem-focused coping. Women saw themselves as having little control over their partners' violence and expressed strong intentions to leave their abusive partners permanently.

Table 1. Means, Standard, Deviations and Range of Obtained Scores

Variable	Mean	Standard Deviation	Range
Physical abuse (CTS-R)	474.04	209.69	135-945
Psychological abuse (PMWI)			
Total	201.99	50.83	80-285
Dominance/isolation	86.39	25.95	31-130
Emotional/verbal	91.39	19.01	33-115
PTSD symptomatology (SCL-90-R)	1.86	.75	.11-3.25
Coping (WCCL-R)			
Emotion focused	59.63	14.31	32-96
Problem focused	28.72	6.77	15-44
Ratio	.50	.12	.25-.92
Perceptions of control	1.98	1.73	1-7
Intention to end relationship	6.23	1.38	2-7

As expected, there was a significant relationship between physical and psychological abuse[2] among our sample of battered women (r [66] = .52, p < .001). Surprisingly, multiple regression analysis results indicated that physical abuse did not account for significant variance in either PTSD symptomatology (R^2 = .02, F [1, 64] = 1.54, ns) or women's intentions to end their abusive relationships (R^2 = .06, F [1, 63] = 3.78, p = .06). On the other hand, psychological abuse was a significant predictor of both PTSD symptomatology (R^2 = .11, F [1, 64] = 8.09, p < .01) and intentions to end the relationship (R^2 = .24, F [1, 63] = 19.40, p < .001), indicating that greater levels of psychological abuse were associated with greater levels of PTSD symptomatology and a greater resolve to leave the abusive partner. When we controlled for the effects of physical abuse by including it as a predictor in the regression equations, psychological abuse continued to account for significant variance in both PTSD symptomatology (full model R^2 = .11; partial R^2 = .09; β = .35, t [63] = 2.52, p < .05) and intention to end the abusive relationship (full model R^2 = .24; partial R^2 = .18; β = .50, t [62] = 3.81, p < .001).

In order to test for the potential moderating effects of PTSD symptomatology on the association between abuse and intentions to terminate the relationship, multiple regressions were conducted separately for physical abuse and for psychological abuse. In each regression, the main effects of abuse and PTSD symptomatology and their interaction (i.e., their product) were entered as predictors of intentions. A significant model with a significant interaction term indicates a significant moderating effect (Baron & Kenny, 1986). PTSD symptomatology proved to be a significant moderator of the effects of both physical (full model R^2 = .15; partial R^2 = .09; β = -1.19, t [61] = -2.57, p = .01) and psychological abuse (full model R^2 = .30; partial R^2 = .05; β = -1.24, t [61] = -2.16, p < .05). In order to examine the moderating effect of PTSD, we computed a median split to create low (< median) and high (≥ median) PTSD symptomatology groups and calculated correlations between abuse and intentions to end the abusive relationship for each of these groups separately. While the relationship between physical abuse and intentions to terminate was significant for women in the low PTSD symptomatology group (r [34] = .54, p = .001), there was no significant relationship for women in the high PTSD symptomatology group (r[32] = -.07, ns). Likewise, psychological abuse and intentions to terminate were highly related among women in the low PTSD symptomatology group (r [33] = .71, p < .001), but there was no significant association for women in the high PTSD symptomatology group (r [32] = .18, ns). Thus, it appeared the presence of high levels of PTSD symptomatology interfered with the intention to leave the abusive partner in response to both physical and psychological abuse.

Because of the significant association between physical and psychological abuse, we conducted a second set of regressions examining the moderating effects of PTSD symptomatology while controlling for the remaining form of abuse. As was the case when we examined main effects, the interaction between PTSD symptomatology and physical abuse was no longer significant after controlling for the effects of psychological abuse. However, the interaction between psychological abuse and PTSD symptomatology continued to be significant even after controlling for physical abuse (full model R^2 = .31; partial R^2 = .06; β = -1.33, t [60] = -2.25, p < .05).

We conducted similar sets of regression analyses to examine potential risk factors for the presence of high levels of PTSD symptomatology in the context of high levels of psychological abuse. The three coping variables (i.e., emotion-focused, problem-focused, and the ratio) and perceptions of control were examined as moderators of the relationship between psychological abuse and PTSD symptomatology in separate regression analyses. Emotion-focused coping and the ratio of emotion- to problem-focused coping strategies were significant predictors of PTSD symptomatology (emotion-focused: R^2 = .13, F [1, 64] = 9.23, p < .01; ratio: R^2 = .07, F [1, 64] = 5.04, p < .05): greater use of emotion-focused coping and greater use of emotion-focused relative to problem-focused coping were associated with greater levels of PTSD symptomatology. While the ratio of emotion- to problem-focused coping strategies was no longer a significant predictor of PTSD symptomatology after controlling for the effects of psychological abuse, emotion-focused coping continued to account for unique variance significantly (t [62] = 2.61, p = .01). However, none of the three coping variables nor perceptions of control moderated the effects of psychological abuse on PTSD symptomatology.

DISCUSSION

The results of the current investigation underscore the importance of assessing and addressing psychological abuse among battered women. Psychological abuse of women was a strong and significant predictor of PTSD symptomatology and intentions to terminate the abusive relationship, accounting for 11% and 24% of the total variance, respectively. More important, the effects of psychological abuse were significant even after controlling for the effects of physical abuse. Surprisingly, physical abuse failed to account significantly for variance in either PTSD symptomatology or intentions to terminate the relationship. All participants in this investigation were battered women residing at emergency shelters. Unlike community samples, our sample was possibly more homogeneous with regard to frequency and severity of physical abuse. Lack of variability in physical abuse scores could make it difficult to obtain significant associations between physical abuse and other variables of interest. However, as reported in Table 1, our sample appeared to be characterized by sufficient variability to detect significant relationships.

Rather than lack of variability, it is possible that our inability to obtain significant results for physical abuse was due to the focus of our measure of physical abuse. Our operationalization of physical abuse was derived by summing the product of frequency and severity of various forms of physical aggression for the year preceding shelter contact. However, women may be more likely to decide to leave their abusers, and/or suffer PTSD symptomatology, in response to the severity of the most recent violent event only and not in response to the cumulative frequency and severity of previous events. For example, a woman who has been slapped and pushed repeatedly during the preceding year and then is assaulted with objects and weapons may be more likely to take initial steps toward leaving her abuser, e.g., reside in a shelter, and may be more committed to terminating the relationship in response to this event than a woman who has been repeatedly threatened and assaulted with objects and weapons and then is slapped and pushed during the most recent violent incident. Alternatively, women may respond to changes in severity and frequency or to their own perceptions of dangerousness rather than absolute, objectively defined levels of frequency and severity.

Although our operationalization of physical abuse may have been consequential, it is also possible that our measure of PTSD symptomatology may have precluded a significant association between PTSD and physical victimization to emerge. PTSD diagnostic criteria are heterogeneous. Foa, Riggs, and Gershuny (1995) suggested that PTSD reactions can consist of three separate but related symptom clusters: numbing, arousal, and intrusion. Further, they suggested that trauma victims may have different psychological reactions characterized by different patterns of PTSD symptoms, and yet all may appropriately be diagnosed as suffering from PTSD. Symptoms of arousal and intrusion were overrepresented by our measure of PTSD symptomatology while symptoms of numbing were underrepresented. Psychological and physical abuse may be related to different pathological reactions such that symptoms from some clusters but not others would be found among survivors of psychological abuse and a different symptom pattern would be found among survivors of physical abuse. If so, additional or alternative measures that adequately assess all types of PTSD symptomatology should be employed in future research. Potential confounding effects of our operationalization of physical abuse and PTSD symptomatology may render it premature to conclude that in future samples physical victimization will not account for PTSD symptomatology or the decision to leave.

While methodological and psychometric factors may have contributed to the inability of physical abuse to predict significantly, the ability of psychological abuse to significantly and independently predict both PTSD symptomatology and intentions to terminate the relationship may reflect that, relative to physical abuse, psychological abuse exerts considerable influence on these variables. First, it is possible that women experienced psychological abuse more frequently than physical abuse. More frequent exposure to psychological abuse may allow it to have a greater impact on women's functioning than the relatively less frequent physical abuse. Unfortunately, our measures of psychological and physical abuse employ response scales of different metric prohibiting direct examination of relative frequency. Second, relative to discreet episodes of physical violence, episodes of psychological abuse may be of longer duration functionally if women internalize psychological abuse, especially emotional abuse and assaults on self-esteem and self-concept such as humiliation. That is, a physically violent episode has a beginning and an end: physically violent acts commence and cease in occurrence during a dispute. Psychological abuse, on the other hand, may be prolonged if events such as name-calling, e.g., "you're crazy/stupid," are incorporated into the self-concept, e.g., "I'm crazy/stupid." Third, psychological assaults and trauma simply may have a greater impact on psychological well-being, at least in regard to PTSD symptomatology, than physical assault. By definition, psychological abuse is psychological in nature. Its targets are affect and cognitions. The specificity and fundamental congruence between psychological abuse and psychological well-being may account for their significant association.

The results of our investigation contribute to the growing empirical base documenting the risk of PTSD among battered women. Participants' mean item score was two times greater than the recommended cutoff score for assessing for clinical levels of PTSD, with 88% of the women scoring above the recommended cutoff score. The women in our investigation completed the assessment within 2 weeks of their arrival at the shelters which, in turn, closely followed an abusive incident, i.e., trauma. The short duration of the period following the trauma (i.e., less than one month) and the absence of standardized clinical assessment do not allow determination of the extent to which women scoring high on our measure of PTSD symptomatology actually would meet DSM-IV criteria (APA, 1994) for the disorder. However, PTSD has been found to be quite prevalent among shelter residents and we would expect a significant proportion of our sample to meet criteria for the disorder as well. Treatment for PTSD symptoms and the disorder *per se* during or after shelter residence should be considered and explored as an appropriate component of intervention.

Neither perceptions of control over the partners' violence nor coping affected the probability that PTSD symptomatology would develop in abusive contexts. However, frequent and preferred use of emotion-focused strategies was predictive of PTSD symptoms. Women who were more likely to rely on ignoring the violence and focusing on less negative aspects of their lives were more likely to develop PTSD symptoms than women who focused on actions that could be taken to reduce, eliminate, or otherwise change the violence and its impact. It is not clear to what extent such action was taken, but it did appear that focusing on potential action buffered women against some of the negative effects of psychological abuse.

While they may not meet clinical criteria, women in our sample reported a high level of distress caused by PTSD symptoms. Of special note, PTSD symptomatology exerted a detrimental impact on women's responses to their victimization: high levels of PTSD symptomatology significantly attenuated the impact of physical abuse and psychological abuse on women's intentions to terminate the abusive relationship. That is, termination of the abusive relationship appeared less likely in the context of PTSD and PTSD-like reactions, apparently, no matter how badly a woman was treated by her partner. Women were able to conceive of termination of the abusive relationship as a viable option and were committed to that option in response to abuse only if they were not hampered by psychological distress. Women experiencing high levels of distress did not appear to be committed to terminating the abusive relationship and should be unlikely to attempt and succeed leaving their abusive partners.

Significant moderation of the main effects of physical and psychological abuse suggests that women's experiences of their own victimization and related decision-making processes may be more complex than we typically assume. Physical and psychological abuse frequency and severity alone did not appear to provide sufficient motivation to disengage from a dangerous situation. Rather, women's psychological well-being determined whether or not abuse was sufficient motivation. Only women who were relatively unscathed psychologically strongly intended to disengage. It may be that when abuse produces significant psychological detriments, women may feel less ready or able to terminate the relationship and attempt self-sufficiency. Interventions with battered women may have to take women's psychological well-being into account before expecting them to choose and attempt self-sufficiency. While women should not be dissuaded from attempting to leave their abusers, supportive services provided may have to vary as a function of women's psychological well-being. Future research should examine directly the extent to which psychological well-being has an impact on women's evaluation of their ability to carry out plans to terminate the relationship and their appraisal of being able to be self-sufficient.

Because of its moderating effects, it seems prudent to attempt to reduce PTSD and related symptoms. The impact of emotion-focused coping suggests that encouraging women to engage in problem-focused coping more frequently, and in preference to the use of emotion-focused strategies, may be productive. In addition to increasing or maintaining psychological distress in the context of abuse, emotion-focused coping may decrease women's ability to stay out of the abusive relationship even if they intend and do carry out plans and strategies for permanently leaving their abusive partners.[3] Continued use of emotion-focused coping may increase the risk of the development of psychological distress in response to the difficulties that may be experienced after leaving the abusive partner such as financial, employment, and housing difficulties. High levels of psychological distress, in turn, may increase the probability of returning to the abusive partner. The results of our investigation, suggesting that coping and distress have a negative impact on women's ability to terminate their abusive relationships, underscore the need for shelter stays that extend beyond the common 30-day limit. Focusing on the development of transitional housing and designing interventions that can be implemented over a longer period of time seem critical. Protective and supportive environments of longer duration would allow women to improve self-esteem, decrease psychological distress, and stabilize their improved affective and cognitive reactions enough to be able to focus on the complex task of independent living. Further, such interventions may increase the probability of maintaining constructive changes and independent living.

NOTES

[1]The overwhelming majority of women indicating "other" specified Baptist or Southern Baptist as their religious affiliations since Baptists traditionally do not consider themselves "Protestant."

[2]There were no differences in the pattern of results as a function of the type of psychological abuse, i.e., dominance/isolation versus emotional/verbal abuse. Further, each type of psychological abuse accounted for significant unique variance in PTSD symptomatology and intentions to terminate the abusive relationship. Accordingly, total PMWI scores were used as the measure of psychological abuse in all analyses.

[3]The association between the use of coping strategies in response to violence and in response to nonviolent, negative relationship events were significant: $r(64) = .72$, $p < .001$, for emotion-focused coping; $r(64) = .59$, $p < .001$, for problem-focused coping. Thus, participants appeared to react similarly to violent and nonviolent stressful events.

REFERENCES

American Psychiatric Association. (1994). *Diagnostic and statistical manual of mental disorders* (4th ed.). Washington, DC: Author.

Aguilar, R. J., & Nightingale, N. N. (1994). The impact of specific battering experiences on the self-esteem of abused women. *Journal of Family Violence, 9,* 35-45.

Arias, I., & Street, A. E. (1996, August). *Children of psychologically abused women: Effects of maternal adjustment and parenting on child outcomes.* Presented at the 8th International Conference on Personal Relationships, Banff, Canada.

Arias, I., Street, A. E., & Brody, G. H. (1996, September). *Depression and alcohol abuse: Women's responses to psychological victimization.* Presented at the American Psychological Association's National Conference on Psychosocial and Behavioral Factors in Women's Health: Research, Prevention, Treatment, and Service Delivery in Clinical and Community Settings. Washington, DC.

Astin, M. C., Lawrence, K. J., & Foy, D. W. (1993). Posttraumatic stress disorder among battered women: Risk and resiliency factors. *Violence and Victims, 8,* 17-28.

Baron, R. M. , & Kenny, D. A. (1986). The moderator-mediator variable distinction in social psychological research: Conceptual, strategic, and statistical considerations. *Journal of Personality and Social Psychology, 51,* 1173-1182.

Cascardi, M., O'Leary, K. D., Lawrence, E. E., & Schlee, K. A. (1995). Characteristics of women physically abused by their spouses and who seek treatment regarding marital conflict. *Journal of Consulting and Clinical Psychology, 63,* 616-623.

Derogatis, L. R. (1977). *SCL-90 administration, scoring and procedure manual for the R(Revised) version.* Johns Hopkins University School of Medicine, Baltimore, MD.

Dutton, D. G., & Hemphill, K. J. (1992). Patterns of socially desirable responding among perpetrators and victims of wife assault. *Violence and Victims, 7,* 29-39.

Foa, E. B., Riggs, D. S., & Gershuny, B. S. (1995). Arousal, numbing, and intrusion: Symptom structure of PTSD following assault. *American Journal of Psychiatry, 152,* 116-120.

Folkman, S., & Lazarus, R. S. (1980). An analysis of coping in a middle-aged community sample. *Journal of Health and Social Behavior, 21,* 219-239.

Folkman, S., & Lazarus, R. S. (1985). If it changes it must be a process: Study of emotion and coping during three stages of a college examination. *Journal of Personality and Social Psychology, 48,* 150-170.

Follingstad, D. R., Rutledge, L. L., Berg, B. J., Hause, E. S., & Polek, D. S. (1990). The role of emotional abuse in physically abusive relationships. *Journal of Family Violence, 5,* 107-120.

Forsythe, C. J., & Compas, B. E. (1987). Interaction of cognitive appraisals of stressful events and coping: Testing the goodness of fit hypothesis. *Cognitive Therapy and Research, 11,* 473-485.

Herbert, T. B., Silver, R. C., & Ellard, J. H. (1991). Coping with an abusive relationship: How and why do women stay? *Journal of Marriage and the Family, 53,* 311-325.

Kahn, F. I., Welch, T. L., & Zillmer, E. A. (1993). MMPI-2 profiles of battered women in transition. *Journal of Personality Assessment, 60,* 100-111.

Kemp, A., Rawlings, E. I., & Green, B. L. (1991). Post-traumatic stress disorder (PTSD) in battered women. *Journal of Traumatic Stress, 4,* 137-148.

Lazarus, R. S., & Folkman, S. (1984). *Stress, appraisal, and coping.* New York: Springer Publishing.

Marshall, L. L. (1996). Psychological abuse of women: Six distinct clusters. *Journal of Family Violence, 11,* 379-409.

Molidor, C. E. (1995). Gender differences of psychological abuse in high school dating relationships. *Child and Adolescent Social Work Journal, 12,* 119-134.

O'Leary, K. D., & Curley, A. D. (1986). Assertion and family violence: Correlates of spouse abuse. *Journal of Marital and Family Therapy, 12,* 281-289.

Parker, B., McFarlane, J., Soeken, K., Torres, S., & Campbell, D. (1993). Physical and emotional abuse in pregnancy: A comparison of adult and teenage women. *Nursing Research, 42,* 173-178.

Ronfeldt, H. M., Bernat, J. A., Arias, I., & Calhoun, K. S. (1996, November). *Peritraumatic reactions and posttraumatic stress disorder among sexually assaulted college women.* Presented at the 30th Annual Convention of the Association for Advancement of Behavior Therapy, New York, NY.

Saunders, B. E., Arata, C. M., & Kilpatrick, D. G. (1990). Development of a crime-related post-traumatic stress disorder scale for women within the Symptom Checklist-90-Revised. *Journal of Traumatic Stress, 3,* 439-448.

Straus, M. A. (1979). Measuring intrafamily conflict and violence: The Conflict Tactics (CT) Scales. *Journal of Marriage and the Family, 41,* 75-88.

Straus, M. A. (1990). The Conflict Tactics Scales and its critics: An evaluation and new data on validity and reliability. In M. A. Straus & R. J. Gelles (Eds.), *Physical violence in American families: Risk factors and adaptations to violence in 8,145 families* (pp. 49-73). New Brunswick, NJ: Transaction Publishers.

Strube, M. J. (1988). The decision to leave an abusive relationship: Empirical evidence and theoretical issues. *Psychological Bulletin, 104,* 236-250.

Tolman, R. M. (1989). The development of a measure of psychological maltreatment of women by their male partners. *Violence and Victims, 4,* 159-177.

Vitanza, S., Vogel, L. C. M., & Marshall, L. L. (1995). Distress and symptoms of posttraumatic stress disorder in abused women. *Violence and Victims, 10,* 23-34.

Walker, L. E. (1984). *The battered woman syndrome.* New York: Springer Publishing.

Chapter 9

Effects of Men's Subtle and Overt Psychological Abuse on Low-Income Women

Linda L. Marshall

My perspective on psychological abuse developed from theories and research on "normal" nonviolent samples from different (sub)disciplines (especially social psychology and communication). This view can best be described as a social influence perspective (Marshall, 1994). Briefly, psychological abuse results from normal intrapersonal and interpersonal processes occurring in everyday interactions. Interpersonal processes can make us feel very good or very bad. These influence processes are the same ones that enable therapists and others to help individuals improve themselves or overcome problems. The abuse is in the effect of an act.

This approach does not discount the effects of obviously abusive controlling or verbally aggressive acts. Indeed, important insights are gained from questionnaires, interaction records, and coding of acts during communication (Babcock, Waltz, Jacobson, & Gottman, 1993; Jacobson, Gottman, Gortner, Burns, & Shortt, 1996; Lloyd, 1996; Vivian & Malone, 1997). I simply propose that the prevailing perspective misses too much that is abusive because many acts can cause psychological and emotional harm. If measures are limited to dominance, obvious control or clear verbal aggression, knowledge will be biased. We will learn a great deal about various forms of aggression in relationships, for example, verbal aggression as it accompanies violent or distressed relationships (Margolin, John, & Gleberman, 1988; Murphy & Cascardi, 1993; O'Leary, Malone, & Tyree, 1994), but little about harm that can be done to women through everyday interactions with men who may or may not have any intent to inflict harm or control their partner.

My social influence approach draws on vast bodies of research (e.g., on anger, attribution, compliance tactics, self-concept, nonverbal behavior, persuasion, expectancy effects, relationship development and dissolution, uncertainty, positive illusions, unintended thought), showing how others often have very strong effects on our attitudes, beliefs, and behaviors without intent, without their awareness, and without our own awareness. In this perspective, the intent of the psychologically abusive act is irrelevant. Thus, an act may be done out of love, to have fun or be playful, or to dominate. Regardless of the intent or the style used, an act may still harm the target and a combination or repetition of messages can cause serious damage. Similarly, the woman's recognition of the act and/or its effects are irrelevant. Social psychology is replete with examples of theories and experiments on many different topics, showing that people often have no awareness that their attitude, belief, behavior, or opinion was influenced by a behavioral induction, characteristics of the situation, or another person's behavior. Thus, there is no need to posit awareness in order to posit effect.

By removing the necessity of considering awareness and intent and by recognizing the potential for everyday interactions to be harmful, it is clear the context must not be restricted to conflict. Although the amount and intensity of conflict, especially in violent relationships, are important and harmful to the relationship and well-being of the individuals, conflictual situations constitute only one portion of communication in relationships. Moreover, statements made during conflicts may be more readily discounted or ignored afterwards as resulting from the heat of the moment. Granted, the statements could still cause hurt feelings which may be long lasting, but the cognitive processing of those statements may be less likely to result in self-questioning than if a hurtful statement was made in a calmer context.

Consider, for example, being told you are fat or ugly, an item on the revised Conflict Tactics Scale (ugly, an item on the revised Conflict Tactics Scale [CTS2]; Straus, Hamby, Boney-McCoy, & Sugarman, 1996). If your partner yelled this during a conflict, it may hurt and you may think about it for a long time, but you could also attribute it to anger or your partner's personality. In contrast, your partner mentions you seem to be putting on weight (or your clothes seem tighter), or your hairstyle could be more attractive. He says he wants everyone to know how beautiful you are and how lucky he is to have you. In this situation, you may be hurt and think about it for a long time, but rather than attributing it to something about the situation or your partner's personality, you are likely to think there is something wrong with you that should be "fixed." If such statements recur, the belief will be strengthened to an extent not likely if such statements only occur as put-downs. Even if your partner told you he was wrong or did not mean to imply you were getting fat, you would still be likely to look at yourself differently. In contrast, you would be less likely to look at yourself differently had he yelled the comment or had said it only when he was in a bad mood.

This example highlights an important distinction that is difficult to describe. Psychological abuse may be obvious, overt, or subtle. Verbal aggression and controlling or dominating acts or statements are examples of obvious acts. Such acts are easily recognizable, readily coded and interpreted as harmful (Babcock et al., 1993; Jacobson et al., 1996; Lloyd, 1996; Vivian & Malone, 1997). An act of psychological abuse would be considered overt when an observer would be able to note the potential for harm and/or the woman would be able to describe the act or resulting feeling with relative ease. Some studies including obvious acts of verbal aggression or control also have measured behaviors which are less clear than obvious acts, but nonetheless overt. Acts may be considered subtle psychological abuse when it would be more difficult for an observer to see the potential for harm, the woman likely would have more difficulty describing the act and her resulting feelings, and/or the act could easily be done in loving and caring ways.

Obvious, overt, and subtle psychological abuse may all result in harm, but the type or locus of harm may differ. Obvious acts may result in anger at the partner and, over time, wear a woman down so she feels overwhelmed. This may be especially likely if the partner is also violent. Obvious acts are likely in distressed relationships and those on their way to the divorce court. Overt acts of psychological abuse may also result in anger and adversely affect a woman's perceptions of her relationship and her partner. Depending on the content of messages, overt acts may harm a woman's well-being in general or in specific areas. However, because subtle acts of psychological abuse are more intangible, they are likely to harm a woman's sense of self and her mental health and well-being more than her perceptions of the relationship and her partner.

Several years ago I conducted an exploratory study of 93 women who had been seriously psychologically abused (Ellington & Marshall, 1997; Marshall, 1994, 1996; Vitanza, Vogel, & Marshall, 1995). The extensive questionnaires and in-depth, semistructured interviews (pilot-tested with 14 women residing in battered women's shelters) were designed to learn more about 40 conceptually distinct categories of psychological abuse listed in Marshall (1994). Verbal aggression was not explored during interviews because it is relatively easy to observe and measure. Symbolic acts of aggression and threats of violence also were not explored during interviews because they are so closely associated with violence that they are usually assessed on the Conflict Tactics Scale (CTS) and the Severity of Violence Scales (Marshall, 1992a; 1992b). Women gave examples and described the effects of 20 to 40 types of psychological abuse during 4-hour interviews.

Transcripts of the interviews made it clear that even types of psychological abuse presumed to be obvious and clearly dominating (e.g., inducing physical debility, showing physical domination) were enacted in loving, joking, or playful ways as well as serious or threatening ways. Further, no male partner used only one style. Even the most violent men did not always inflict psychological abuse with an aggressive or dominating style. Men were often very gentle and loving when they enacted behaviors in the various categories of psychological abuse. Thus, the importance of assessing both subtle and overt psychological abuse was underscored.

As noted by O'Leary and Jouriles (1994), we must begin to disentangle the effects of psychological abuse and physical violence. In addition, sexual aggression is another harmful (Campbell, Miller, Cardwell, & Belknap, 1994; Kilpatrick, Best, Saunders, & Veronen, 1988) but understudied form of abuse in intimate relationships (Crowell & Burgess, 1996). This study expands Marshall (1996) examining the effects of subtle and overt psychological abuse, violence, and sexual aggression on women's emotional state and relationship perceptions. Violence, overt psychological abuse, and/or sexual aggression by a male partner may affect women's self esteem (Arias, Lyons, & Street, 1997; Campbell et al., 1994; Cascardi & O'Leary, 1992; Follingstad, Rutledge, Berg, Hause, & Polek, 1990; Pipes & LeBov-Keeler, 1997; Sommers & Check, 1987; Stets, 1991), stress (Campbell, 1989; Cascardi & Vivian, 1995; Dutton, 1992; Marshall & Rose, 1990), health (Barnett & Hamberger, 1992; Bergman & Brismar, 1991; Campbell, 1989; Cascardi, Langhrinsen, & Vivian, 1992; Riggs, Kilpatrick, & Resnick, 1992; Stuart & Campbell, 1989), emotional distress (Arias et al., 1997; Campbell, 1989; Campbell et al., 1994; Kilpatrick et al., 1988), and risk of suicide (Gondolf, Fisher, & McFerron, 1990; Kurz & Stark, 1989; Stuart & Campbell, 1989). These effects harm women's emotional, cognitive, and physical state. These same types of abuse have been shown to affect perceptions women have about their relationship and their partner. For example, the quality of women's relationship (e.g., satisfaction, distress) is affected by violence and verbal aggression (Arias et al., 1997; Barnett & Hamberger, 1992; Frieze & McHugh, 1992; Kasian & Painter, 1992; O'Leary et al., 1994) as is women's fear (Kilpatrick et al., 1988; Jacobson, Gottman, Waltz, Rushe, Babcock, & Holtzworth-Munroe, 1994; Kelly & DeKeseredy, 1994; Saunders, 1996). In fact, even in nonviolent relationships, women fear their partner's verbal aggression (i.e., saying nasty things) as found by O'Leary and Jouriles (1994) in a re-analysis of an earlier study. If several obvious and subtle types of abuse are included in more studies, different types of effects may become evident.

Too little is known about subtle and overt forms of psychological abuse to make specific predictions but general trends were expected. Women are likely to recognize their partner's dominating, controlling, and aggressive behavior. Therefore, men's overt psychological abuse, violence, and sexual aggression were expected to affect the perceptions women had about their partner and relationship. Based on past research, these forms of aggression would also be likely to affect women's intrapersonal state. However, based on the social influence literature and the conceptualization described here, it was likely that subtle psychological abuse would have more of an effect on women's state and well-being than the other three forms of partner abuse. The exception was that perception of physical health would be more affected by violence and sexual aggression than by either type of psychological abuse because of the potential for physical harm from these acts.

This study is part of a longitudinal project examining the effects of psychological abuse, violence, and sexual aggression on low-income women. Understanding these women is important for several reasons. Unless income is attenuated, ethnicity and socioeconomic status are likely to be confounded. In general, poverty is associated with poor physical and mental health. These effects may be exacerbated if women's vulnerability is increased by any type of partner abuse. In addition, women of lower socioeconomic status are more at risk than middle-class women for domestic violence (Mihalic & Elliott, 1997; Zawitz, 1994) and harm (Stuart & Campbell, 1989), homelessness (Brice-Baker, 1994; Shinn, Knickman, & Weitzman, 1991; Wood, Valdez, Hayashi, & Shen, 1990) and killing their partner (Roberts, 1996) as a result of domestic violence. Further, women who sustain partner violence use medical and other resources more than those in nonviolent relationships (Bergman & Brismar, 1991; Cascardi et al., 1992), especially if they are poor (McClosky, 1996). Low-income women must rely on public resources which may or may not be responsive to their needs which result from their partner's behavior (Kurz & Stark, 1989). The ultimate goal of the larger study is to identify points at which intervention could be of most benefit to women and to identify likely resources that could provide effective, ethnically appropriate intervention. Therefore, it was necessary to have a broad-based sample of ethnically diverse women who had and had not sustained violence from their partner at the beginning of the study.

METHOD

Sample

The data reported here are from the first of seven waves of interviews in a longitudinal study. Women were recruited through newspaper articles, personal encounters (e.g., on the street, in businesses, at health fairs or their homes), flyers (in businesses, libraries, churches), and by referral from participants over the course of 20 months. This study, Project HOW: Health Outcomes of Women, was described as focusing on factors that harm and help women's health. To schedule an interview, women had to be in a long-term (at least 1 year) heterosexual relationship, between the ages of 20 and 47 years, and live within 175% of poverty or be receiving public aid. The age range was chosen to correspond to census categories and to encompass ages at which relationship violence may increase and decrease. The purpose of limiting household income was to keep ethnicity from being confounded with class and to ensure that most women in the study would need to rely on public resources for help. Federal poverty tables were used to cross-tabulate income from work and number of people in the household unless women were receiving Aid to Families with Dependent Children (AFDC), food stamps, or a rent subsidy.[1] There was no requirement regarding the presence or absence of violence or any other type of abuse.

Of the 998 women who began the first interview, 164 were found not to qualify. During the interviews it was often discovered that their relationship was not ongoing with close contact (e.g., their partner was in prison, or they were married but separated). These interviews were not completed. The second primary reason for disqualification was income. Women were asked about their household income and the number of people supported by that income during screening, but many apparently determined the amount more exactly before their interview. Consequently, they reported more money during interviews than during screening. These women were dropped after their interview. All women were paid $15 in cash and received a tote bag and T-shirt with the project logo.

Of the 834 women in the study, 303 (36.3%) were African Americans, 271 (32.5%) were Euro-Americans, and 260 (31.2%) were Mexican Americans. The mean age of women was 32.81 years. Participants were seriously dating (24.1%), cohabiting (12.8%), in a self-defined common-law marriage (21.7%), or legally married (41.4%) to their partner. The duration of these relationships ranged from 1 to 33 years ($M = 7.70$ years).

Instruments

Women were interviewed in one of two storefront offices in the geographical area targeted for the study. The mean length of the structured interviews was 2.5 hours. Trained undergraduate females conducted the interviews. The results reported here are from measures of psychological abuse, physical and sexual aggression by women's partner, women's personal characteristics and emotional state at the time of the interview, and factors reflective of and related to their relationship. The state and relationship measures chosen for this study assessed constructs likely to affect women's overall sense of well-being. Pilot testing with a similar population resulted in revising, simplifying wording, and modifying ratings scales.

Violence and Sexual Aggression. The Severity of Violence Against Women Scale (SVAWS; Marshall, 1992a) was used to assess acts of violence and sexual aggression women sustained from their partner. Nineteen of the 46 items assess threats of violence which were not used in this study because of the high correlation

($r = .85$) with acts of violence. Twenty-one items assessed physical aggression, ranging from relatively minor acts (e.g., holding women down, pinning them in place, grabbing suddenly or forcefully), through acts classified as mild and moderate, to severe acts which could cause serious injury or death (e.g., use of a club-like object, beat up). Six items measured sexual aggression by the partner (e.g., physically forced to have sex, made to have anal sex against her will). Women reported the perceived number of times their partner had done each act during their entire relationship on 6-point rating scales (0 = never, 1 = once, 5 = a great many times). The internal consistency of the violence ($\alpha = .95$) and sexual aggression ($\alpha = .85$) scales were quite high.

Psychological Abuse. My earlier study showed that items to measure both overt and subtle psychological abuse must allow enactment to occur with a broad range of styles and message content areas (Marshall, 1994, 1996). Items were written so women would recognize the act whether it was done in a loving style (e.g., I love you so much that I hate to see you so upset by your family; it's too bad you see them so often), a dominating or controlling style, and/or a teasing or joking style. This was done with more success for some items (e.g., made you feel guilty) than others (e.g., yell at you). In addition, the content of items representing a partner's messages had to be less specific than items used in past research to allow relevance to a broad range of women.

Women were told "Both men and women do these kinds of things, but this time we want your partner's behavior. Some things may be nice and others may be unpleasant. Men may do these acts in a loving way, a joking way, or a serious way." Women rated the 184 items on 10-point frequency scales anchored by "never" and "almost daily." The elimination of items began when results from about two-thirds of the sample were available. It was important to have broadly relevant scales that were independent of whether or not women were battered, but it was also important to have items that were neither too common nor too uncommon. Consequently, items that were endorsed by more than about half the women were eliminated as were those endorsed by fewer than 15%. Used here are the initial versions of the Men's Psychological-Harm and Abuse in Relationships Measure-Overt scales and -Subtle scales (MP-HARM-O and MP-HARM-S; Marshall & Guarnaccia, 1998).

For present purposes, factor analysis with orthogonal rotation was conducted on the 35 items representing overt and the 33 items representing subtle psychological abuse. The number of factors to use for each scale (overt and subtle) was determined by examination of the eigen values, scree plots, and cross-loads. In addition to the empirical criteria (i.e., a gap in eigen value, flattening of the scree plot, and less than 2.5% of the variance accounted for by a factor), the factors were also examined for conceptual logic. (Results of the factor analyses are available from the author.) Representative items for the factors are listed in Table 1.

Factor analysis was first conducted on the 35 items indicative of overt psychological abuse. Although four items cross-loaded, the four factor solution resulted in interpretable, completely uncorrelated factors ($r = .00$). Factor 1, Dominate,

Table 1. Examples of Abbreviated Psychological Abuse Items

Overt Psychological Abuse

Dominate	try to get you to say you were wrong even if you think you were right
	tell you something he did was your fault
	remind you of times he was right and you were wrong
	try to get you to apologize for something that wasn't your fault
	use an offensive or hurtful tone
	get angry or hurt if you talk about him or your relationship
	make you feel like nothing you say will have an effect
	make you feel like you can't keep up with changes in what he wants
Indifference	act like you don't matter
	ignore you
	use money you need or keep money from you when you need it
	avoid you
Monitor	check to see if you're doing what you said you would be doing
	check up on you
	act like he doesn't believe you
	try to keep you from seeing friends or family
Discredit	tell others you have emotional problems or are crazy
	tell you friends or family don't care about you
	tell you what he likes about you then get upset about the same thing
	tell others things that make you look bad

Subtle Psychological Abuse

Undermine	make you worry about your physical health and well-being
	make you worry about whether you could take care of yourself
	make you worry about your emotional health and well-being
	make you feel ashamed of yourself
	get you to question yourself, making you feel insecure and less confident
	make you feel guilty about something you have or haven't done
	say his hurtful actions were good for you or will make you a better person
Discount	act secretive or try to keep things from you
	do things that make you feel small, less than what you were
	discourage from interests he is not part of
	do or say something that harms your self-respect or pride in yourself
	act like you can do what you want then become upset if you do
	act like there is something wrong with you mentally/emotionally
Isolate	discourage you from talking to his family, friends, or people he knows
	make it difficult to go somewhere or talk to someone
	point out he is the only one who really understands you
	discourage you from having your own friends
	keep you from having time for yourself
	try to keep you from showing feelings

consisted of 17 items representing overt attempts to dominate and control a woman. This factor accounted for 59.8% of the variance. Factor 2, Indifference, consisted of 5 items and accounted for 3.5% of the variance. Factor 3, Monitor, consisted of 6 items and accounted for 3% of the variance. Factor 4, Discredit, consisted of 7 items and accounted for 2.6% of the variance. The factor scores, which together accounted for 69% of the total variance, were used in analyses.

Factor analysis was then conducted on the 33 items representing subtle acts of psychological abuse. The three-factor solution was most clearly interpretable although two items cross-loaded. Factor 1, Undermine, consisted of 12 items and accounted for 61.4% of the variance. Factor 2, Discount, consisted of 11 items and accounted for 3.3% of the variance. Factor 3, Isolate, consisted of 10 items and accounted for 3% of the variance. The factor scores, which together accounted for 67.7% of the total variance, were used in analyses.

Women's State. The measures used to assess women's state covered a range of constructs related to well-being. Self-esteem was measured with Rosenberg's (1965) 10-item scale. This is the most widely used brief instrument available with adequate comparative data for ethnically diverse women. Women rated the accuracy of statements on 7-point scales anchored by "completely false," "I'm never like this" to "completely true," "exactly like me." Despite the modification in ratings, the scale was internally consistent ($\alpha = .83$).

Cohen, Kamarck, and Mermelstein's (1983) 14-item measure assessed how well women were handling stress. This is a general measure of perceived stress, with items reflecting difficulty in coping (e.g., felt nervous and stressed; been upset because of something that happened unexpectedly; felt difficulties were piling up so high that you could not overcome them). Responses were made on 7-point scales ranging from never (1) through about half the time (4) to always (7). Internal consistency was adequate ($\alpha = .76$).

Perception of physical health was measured with a slightly modified item developed by Hays, Sherbourne, and Mazel (1993). Women were asked to "Rate your overall quality of life in terms of your health. A zero is the worst possible and 10 is the best possible health quality of life." The item was in a section of the interview devoted to physical health (e.g., seeing a physician, health insurance, health conditions).

The Symptom Checklist 90 (Derogatis, Lipman, & Covi, 1973) assessed women's overall emotional distress. Both the SCL90 and SCL90-R are widely used with clinical and nonclinical samples. Women rated how much they had been bothered by each symptom during the past month on 5-point scales (not at all, a little bit, moderately, quite a bit, extremely). Internal consistency on the global distress scale was high ($\alpha = .98$).

Battered women may be at risk for suicide so a measure of severe depression or suicidal ideation was needed. Goldberg and Hillier's (1979) General Health Questionnaire is a multidimensional measure of emotional health. Five items reflecting severe depression and suicidal ideation were modified because the measure was developed for use with British samples. The items asked how often women felt that life is entirely hopeless; felt that life isn't worth living; thought of the possibility that you might do away with yourself; found yourself wishing you were dead and away from it all; found that the idea of taking your own life kept coming into your mind. Items were rated on 7-point scales ranging from never (1) through about half the time (4) to always (7). The scale was internally consistent (a = .92).

Relationship-Related Measures. Two items measured women's fear of their partner's violence. Women were asked how many times they were afraid they might be seriously injured and afraid they might be killed using the same 6-point rating scale as used for the SVAWS (never to a great many times). Only 707 women were asked these questions. (Some early interviewers did not ask these questions unless women had been injured by their partner but the questions were supposed to be asked of every woman who had sustained any threat or act of violence.) This index had strong internal consistency ($\alpha = .88$).

Cloven and Roloff (1991) found that rumination about relationship conflicts was associated with the severity of the conflicts. (In turn, rumination has been associated with depression according to Nolen-Hoeksema, 1987.) A 5-item measure assessing women's rumination about problems in their relationship and with their partner was based on Cloven and Roloff's measure of mulling. The items assessed how much women thought about those problems; worried about those problems; how thoughts of those problems affected their daily activities; amount of effort they put into examining or evaluating those problems; and time they spent considering and thinking about those problems. The 7-point rating scale was anchored by "not at all" and "extremely much." This scale also showed strong internal consistency ($\alpha = .88$).

The measure of marital well-being used here (Acitelli, Douvan, & Veroff, 1989) has been used longitudinally with an ethnically diverse sample (Acitelli, Douvan, & Veroff, 1997; Crohan & Veroff, 1989; Hatchett, Veroff, & Douvan, 1995). The item addressing overall satisfaction was replaced with an item measuring stability. The six items (Taking things together, how happy is your relationship; When you think about your relationship, what each of you puts into it and gets out of it, how happy do you feel; How certain are you that you will be together one year from now; What about 5 years from now; How stable is your relationship; In the past 6 months, how often have you considered leaving him) were rated on 7-point scales ("not at all or never" to "completely or extremely often"). This brief scale was internally consistent ($\alpha = .92$).

RESULTS[2]

Many community samples contain few women who are battered to a degree comparable to those who enter shelters. To obtain a profile for this sample, the SVAWS violence subscales were used to classify women based on the most serious act of violence they had sustained from their partner. Table 2 shows a nearly equal proportion of women were with completely nonviolent partners as were with men who had inflicted severe, potentially life-threatening violence. Just under a third of the sample were at each extreme. The table also shows the mean frequency score (i.e., the sum of the 20 acts of violence) associated with each level of violence.

First, zero order correlations were calculated among the types of abuse, although multiple regression procedures are robust for multicollinearity. (Correlations nearing .80 may be acceptable in samples this large; Berry & Feldman, 1985.) Table 3 shows these correlations. Most correlations were less than .40. Only two correlations are moderately high; between overt Factor 2, Indifference, and subtle Factor 2, Discount, and between violence and sexual aggression. Then 9 multiple regressions were calculated allowing each type of abuse to enter in order of importance to explain the variance in women's state (self-esteem, stress, health quality, emotional distress, severe depression, and suicidal ideation) and relationship (fear, rumination about problems, quality, duration) well-being. Abuse consisted of direct aggression (violence, sexual aggression), the overt (dominate, being indifferent, monitor, discredit) and subtle (undermine, discount, isolate) psychological abuse factors. Explanatory variables are reported in order of appearance.

Table 2. Distribution by Worst Act of Violence Sustained

	Percent in category	Range of scores	Mean score
No violent acts	31.5		
Acts of minor violence	16.2	1 to 14	2.27
Acts of mild violence	10.4	1 to 18	5.39
Acts of moderate violence	10.8	1 to 32	6.80
Acts of severe violence	31.1	1 to 99	21.05

Table 3. Correlations Among Predictor Variables

	Aggression		Psychological Abuse					
			Overt				Subtle	
	1	2	3	4	5	6	7	8
1. violent acts								
2. sexual aggression	.55							
3. overt-Dominate	.29	.23						
4. overt-Indifference	.36	.26	..					
5. overt-Monitor	.26	.24	..	..				
6. overt-Discredit	.25	.29	..	..	..			
7. subtle-Undermine	.30	.30	.35	.27	..	.36		
8. subtle-Discount	.35	.25	.36	.56	.31	..	..	
9. subtle-Isolate	.35	.33	.25	..	.38	.46	..	..

The *n* for each correlation ranged between 822 and 834. Correlations are *p* < .000.

The subtle psychological abuse factors emerged most often to explain the variance in women's state. Subtle Undermining (beta = -.357), Discounting (beta = -.126), and Isolation (beta = -.149) combined with overt Indifference (beta = -.098) to help explain women's self-esteem, $R = .46$, $p < .0001$. Subtle Undermining (beta = -.199), Discounting (beta = -.141), and Isolating (beta = -.128) helped explain health quality of life in this sample, $R = .27$, $p < .0001$. Similarly, subtle Undermining (beta = .388), Isolation (beta = .266), and Discounting (beta = .216) combined with overt Monitoring (beta = .073) emerged for global emotional distress, $R = .55$, $p < .0001$. Women's severe depression and suicidal ideation score was partially explained by subtle Undermining (beta = .308), Isolation (beta = .170) and Discounting (beta = .117) as well as sexual aggression (beta = .077) by their partner, $R = .41$, $p < .0001$. In contrast, overtly Dominating (beta = .250), Indifference (beta = .225), Discrediting (beta = .105), and Monitoring (beta = .109) acts as well as subtle Undermining (beta = .078) were significant predictors of women's stress, $R = .41$, $p < .0001$.

Although overt psychological abuse was expected to be more important for relationship variables, subtle acts again appeared to have more effect. Much of the variance in the index representing women's fear of severe injury or death at the hands of their partner was explained by men's violence (beta = .528) with significant contributions by overt Monitoring (beta = .090) and subtle Undermining (beta = .117), Isolation (beta = .100), and Discounting (beta = .076), $R = .67$, $p < .0001$. Women ruminated about problems as their partner subtly Undermined (beta = .314), Discounted (beta = .290), and Isolated (beta = .214) them, $R = .48$, $p < .0001$. Relationship quality was partially explained by subtle Discounting (beta = -.428), Isolation (beta = -.236), and Undermining (beta = -.204) as well as overt Indifference (beta = -.085) and violence (beta = -.080), $R = .63$, $p < .0001$. Finally, the duration of women's relationship was partially explained by overt Indifference (beta = .131), less subtle Isolation (beta = -.168), overtly Dominating acts (beta = .102) and sexual aggression (beta = .095), $R = .24$, $p < .0001$.

Additional Analyses

Although the various types of psychological abuse were expected to make significant contributions in the regression equations, violence and sexual aggression were expected to emerge much more often and be more important than was found. Further, subtle psychological abuse emerged much more consistently than overt psychological abuse which conflicts with the extant literature. Consequently, a series of hierarchical regression equations was calculated to confirm that subtle psychological abuse was, indeed, as important as it appeared.

In the first series of equations, men's violence and sexual aggression were entered at Step 1. The four types of overt psychological abuse were entered at Step 2 before the three types of subtle psychological abuse were entered at Step 3. This procedure stacks the deck against subtle psychological abuse. If subtle psychological abuse accounted for a significant amount of the variance even after controlling for men's direct aggression and overt psychological abuse, it would support the notion that acts which cannot be readily identified as harmful do indeed take their toll on women. In the second series of equations, the subtle psychological abuse factors were entered at Step 1, followed by overt psychological abuse at Step 2. Finally, men's direct aggression (violence and sexual aggression) was entered at Step 3.

In most community samples, violence scores would be less likely than more normally distributed variables (in this case overt and subtle psychological abuse) to make a significant contribution using these hierarchical procedures. This is because most of the violence in such samples is relatively minor with relatively low scores. Table 2 showed that was not an issue for this sample because over 30% had sustained severe, potentially life-threatening violence. The level of violence sustained by so many women in this study is likely similar to samples drawn from police reports, emergency rooms, and shelters. Moreover, all women were relatively poor when their data were collected. That, also, suggests that a reasonably large proportion is, in several ways, similar to samples of identified battered women.

The purpose of the hierarchical regressions was to confirm the results which indicated that subtle psychological abuse was generally more harmful than either overt psychological abuse or direct aggression. On the other hand, the procedures must be considered exploratory because this was the first study to examine all these different types of partner abuse together in such a systematic way. Consequently, the results are important to develop theory and hypotheses. As with Jacobson and associates' study (1996), alpha was not adjusted for the 18 regression equations.

To facilitate comparisons, the results from both series are presented side by side in Table 4. First, in eight of the nine equations the subtle psychological abuse factors made a small but significant contribution even when they were entered last, after the other types of abuse. Despite the appearance that violence and sexual aggression made major contributions to the state and relationship variables in the first series (on the left), these effects were sufficiently strong to make a significant contribution in only 2 (fear and relationship duration) of the 9 equations when they were entered last (on the right). The *R* at Step 1 was higher on the right side of the table when subtle abuse was entered, except in the equations for fear. Further, in all but one instance overt psychological abuse made a significant unique contribution when scores were entered after men's direct aggression, but nonsignificant in four of the nine equations when it followed subtle psychological abuse.

DISCUSSION

The results clearly show that an expanded view of psychological abuse is warranted. Surprisingly, the subtle forms of psychological abuse had an effect more frequently than overt psychological abuse, violence, or sexual aggression, regardless of whether intrapersonal or relationship measures were being examined.

Table 4. Hierarchical Regression

Variables Entered	R	R^2chg	pchg	Variables Entered	R	R^2chg	pchg
Self-Esteem							
Step 1 Aggression	.25	.064	.0001	Step 1 Subtle	.45	.202	.0001
Step 2 Overt	.41	.105	.0001	Step 2 Overt	.46	.010	.05
Step 3 Subtle	.46	.047	.0001	Step 3 Aggression	.47	.004	ns
Stress							
Step 1 Aggression	.29	.083	.0001	Step 1 Subtle	.41	.169	.0001
Step 2 Overt	.41	.087	.0001	Step 2 Overt	.42	.007	ns
Step 3 Subtle	.42	.008	.05	Step 3 Aggression	.42	.003	ns
Health Quality of Life							
Step 1 Aggression	.19	.037	.0001	Step 1 Subtle	.27	.075	.0001
Step 2 Overt	.26	.030	.0001	Step 2 Overt	.28	.004	ns
Step 3 Subtle	.28	.013	.01	Step 3 Aggression	.28	.001	ns
Global Emotional Distress							
Step 1 Aggression	.36	.130	.0001	Step 1 Subtle	.54	.295	.0001
Step 2 Overt	.53	.151	.0001	Step 2 Overt	.55	.008	ns
Step 3 Subtle	.55	.023	.0001	Step 3 Aggression	.55	.002	ns
Severe Depression and Suicidal Ideation							
Step 1 Aggression	.30	.089	.0001	Step 1 Subtle	.41	.166	.0001
Step 2 Overt	.40	.071	.0001	Step 2 Overt	.42	.011	.03
Step 3 Subtle	.43	.022	.0001	Step 3 Aggression	.43	.005	ns
Fear of Severe Injury or Death							
Step 1 Aggression	.64	.414	.0001	Step 1 Subtle	.49	.243	.0001
Step 2 Overt	.66	.028	.0001	Step 2 Overt	.51	.013	.04
Step 3 Subtle	.67	.003	ns	Step 3 Aggression	.67	.189	.0001
Rumination About Relationship and Partner							
Step 1 Aggression	.30	.088	.0001	Step 1 Subtle	.48	.228	.0001
Step 2 Overt	.47	.136	.0001	Step 2 Overt	.48	.006	ns
Step 3 Subtle	.48	.009	.03	Step 3 Aggression	.48	.000	ns
Relationship Quality							
Step 1 Aggression	.42	.180	.0001	Step 1 Subtle	.62	.386	.0001
Step 2 Overt	.62	.207	.0001	Step 2 Overt	.63	.012	.003
Step 3 Subtle	.63	.016	.0001	Step 3 Aggression	.63	.004	ns
Relationship Duration							
Step 1 Aggression	.10	.011	.02	Step 1 Subtle	.17	.029	.0001
Step 2 Overt	.25	.050	.0001	Step 2 Overt	.24	.028	.0001
Step 3 Subtle	.26	.009	.05	Step 3 Aggression	.27	.013	.004

Aggression consists of violence and sexual aggression scores. Overt consists of the four factor scores (Dominate, Indifference, Monitor, Discredit) for overt psychological abuse. Subtle consists of the three factor scores (Undermine, Discount, Isolate) for subtle psychological abuse.

As dictated by my approach to psychological abuse, there was little association between acts of physical or sexual aggression and psychological abuse. The correlations were generally low. The highest correlations between direct aggression and psychological abuse was only .36 (physical violence and overt indifference). The correlations suggest that suffering one form of abuse from a partner will not necessarily increase the likelihood of sustaining other forms of abuse. However, other researchers have found significant and sizable correlations between psychological and physical abuse (Straus et al., 1996).

Overall, the three types of subtle psychological abuse emerged more often to predict outcomes than did the four types of overt psychological abuse, violence, and sexual aggression. Even when the dependent variable was women's fear of injury or death as a result of their partner's violence, subtle and overt psychological abuse made independent contributions. The results of the two series of hierarchical multiple regression were even more impressive. Not only did subtle psychological abuse account for significant variance after controlling for men's violence, sexual aggression, and overt psychological abuse, but it almost completely eliminated the effects of the other types of abuse when it was entered first on most measures.

It is not illogical that subtle psychological abuse would have broad effects. Enactment of the relevant items in Table 1 would likely cause a woman to feel uncertain about herself, unimportant and tentative during interactions with others. If uncertainty or discrepancies in a woman's sense of self were created or reinforced, the effects could be pervasive (Trope & Liberman, 1996). The woman may begin to view herself differently, for example, by mistrusting her perceptions. Processes (e.g., attributions, rumination, behavior change, expectancy effects) would be set in motion which are likely to result in confirming the problematic self-perceptions. Thus, many aspects of women's life could be affected by a partner who simply raised issues that created or reinforced a woman's personal vulnerabilities.

Of all the types of abuse, a man subtly undermining his partner emerged as a strong predictor most consistently. Apparently, having one's sense of self weakened results in the broadest effects. A sense of self is central to factors associated with personal well-being and is important for judgments about one's relationship. It is likely that most aspects of life could be affected if a woman did not believe in herself or trust her own perceptions. This type of psychological abuse always emerged in the logical direction.

Having been discounted or subtly isolated, the second and third subtle psychological abuse factors also emerged more often than overt psychological abuse or direct aggression for both women's state and relationship. When they were important, their contribution was in the logical direction. A partner enacting behaviors represented by the discount subscale could make a woman feel unimportant. If a woman felt insignificant, especially in her primary relationship, it could be very difficult for her to believe she was important in other parts of her own life or in the lives of others.

It should be noted that the subtle factor isolation is somewhat different than usually discussed in the partner violence literature. Most investigators have tended to conceptualize isolation as being done in very obvious ways. It has been thought of as a batterer keeping his partner away from others or making it difficult for her to communicate with others (e.g., restricting her use of a car or the telephone). Isolation in this study is more akin to alienation or psychological distance from others and even from oneself (e.g., somehow keep you from having time for yourself). Sustaining this type of subtle psychological abuse could result in a woman feeling as if she were alone or different from others even if she has a wide circle of friends. It could also keep her from enjoying the small, private pleasures most women enjoy (e.g., taking a long, hot bath).

The very nature of subtle psychological abuse would make it difficult to terminate and to treat, especially if acts appeared to be done out of love and concern for the woman rather than aggressively for purposes of control. It would be very difficult for both the woman and her therapist to recognize either that these acts were occurring or that these acts were causing emotional harm directly or through other intrapersonal or interpersonal processes. It may be that women who have endured subtle psychological abuse often seek therapy for symptoms caused by the abuse, but the likelihood that a partner's acts would be implicated as possible causal factors by the woman or her therapist is small. Further, from a social influence perspective, the woman would be unable to gain or maintain psychological and emotional well-being as long as her partner inflicted the subtle abuse.

Altogether, the types of overt psychological abuse also emerged more frequently than violence and sexual aggression. At first glance, it is difficult to imagine overt psychological abuse being done in a loving way, but both forms (i.e., subtle and overt) conceivably could be done in loving, joking, serious, and aggressive ways, except perhaps indifference. Thus, these acts may also be difficult to recognize but if alert to the possibility, the potential for harm inherent in the acts could be recognized by an observer or the woman herself. It is this characteristic of acts that make the label overt psychological abuse appropriate. In comparison to subtle acts, with overt acts it would be relatively easy to see the partner's behavior as one cause of associated symptoms.

Of the different types of overt abuse, monitoring and indifference emerged more often than dominating and discrediting. Overt types of psychological abuse were not more likely to be associated with relationship variables than with women's current physical and emotional state. Overall, overt psychological abuse may have the most effect indirectly by increasing women's perceived stress or decreasing their confidence in handling stressful events. Stress, then, may affect other aspects of women's well-being.

The most surprising finding for overt psychological abuse was the relatively little impact of the dominating factor, given its centrality in the partner violence literature. It only emerged twice. Both dominating and monitoring can be thought of as controlling behaviors, especially if done in serious or aggressive ways.

Therefore, these factors are most similar to the way psychological abuse is usually addressed in the literature. There are several intriguing possibilities.

If dominating and monitoring actually have so little direct impact on women, programs and therapy for batterers and battered women may be focusing too much time and effort on something that is comparatively benign. It may be that most women are able to dismiss these types of acts as something about their partner that they have to put up with. In this case, men's behavior would be attributed to the men, not to women's own personality or behavior. For some women it may not be too bothersome, whereas it may eventually cause others to terminate the relationship. Thus, one reason why these controlling types of psychological abuse had so little effect could be that most women tend to leave men who dominate them or monitor their behavior.

On the other hand, with only four types of overt psychological abuse measured in this study, other overt and obvious acts of dominance or control are not precluded from having adverse effects on women. It must be remembered that the acts were not necessarily done in an aggressive, hostile, or possessive way. The partners of some women may enact the behaviors in a style or with specific messages that are congruent with traditional research and treatment, whereas others may enact the behaviors in very different ways. Alternatively, dominating or controlling acts may have serious effects only in the presence of a specific combination of factors in the relationship. Before concluding that controlling acts are not particularly harmful, research must combine the traditional approach to psychological abuse with the approach taken here.

There was a moderate correlation between overt indifference and subtle discounting. Examination of the items in Table 1 shows that both factors have elements of withdrawal or interpersonal distance. The overlap may reflect an underlying category of psychological abuse, perhaps withdrawal or rejection (Marshall, 1994). On the other hand, the relationship is not strong. It is possible that overt indifference occurs in most relationships that are in the process of dissolution as well as those that are psychologically abusive or distressed. In contrast, subtle discounting may be less likely to occur in dissolving relationships because there is also an element of commitment. For example, outside interests may be encouraged, rather than discouraged, in withdrawing, distancing, or divorcing couples.

The results are relative, not absolute. It is not that overt psychological abuse and direct aggression had little effect. Rather, in comparison to the effects of subtle psychological abuse, the effects of overt psychological abuse as well as violence and sexual aggression are relatively less likely and often weaker. Examination of the left side of Table 4 shows that overt psychological abuse significantly contributes to the explanation of the measures used in this study. Moreover, the unique contribution is often relatively large, even after the effects of direct aggression are controlled. Thus, even in the presence of direct aggression, overt psychological abuse is relatively harmful. In contrast, the right side of the table shows that overt psychological abuse makes relatively little contribution when the effects of subtle psychological abuse are controlled. Thus, in the presence of subtle psychological abuse, overt psychological abuse may do relatively little harm.

Neither violence nor sexual aggression contributed as much to the outcome measures as expected, but they were not unimportant. When either emerged with a significant contribution, its value usually decreased when any form of psychological abuse entered the equations. The primary (and logical) exception was on women's fear for their physical well-being. These results and the hierarchical procedures support anecdotal evidence from battered women who have said the psychological abuse was worse than the violence. The difference is that the most harmful psychological abuse was not of the dominating and controlling type that has been assumed. However, more research including the different forms of abuse is needed before conclusions can be drawn about these issues.

Because all women lived below or near the federal poverty level, the results may not generalize to women of higher economic status. Due to economic realities, more women in this study than in other studies may have too few alternatives to remaining with an abusive man. They, therefore, may be forced to make a stronger effort to effectively cope with abuse than would women with more economic resources. For example, it could be that violence and sexual aggression so rarely had an effect because these women were highly motivated to protect themselves from the harmful effects in order to remain with their partner for economic reasons. However, the likelihood that women's motivation to remain in their relationship could account for the relative lack of effect of obvious abuse (overt psychological abuse, violence, and sexual aggression) in comparison to subtle forms of abuse is not greater for two reasons. First, women who live in or close to poverty may be slightly better off financially in terms of eligibility for various types of public aid if they do not have a partner. (If so, this could change after all welfare reforms are fully implemented.) In addition, women willing to report domestic violence are exempt from some of the welfare reform limitations. Therefore, low-income women may be less motivated to stay with an abusive man than middle-class women whose economic status would decrease by loss of a partner's income. The second reason relates to the complexity of ties in the relationship which may be reflected in women's choice of terms for their relationship. Although 63% were married (common-law and legal), 24% of the sample were only dating their partner. Of the 288 women who were cohabiting, 37% did not consider themselves to be in a common-law marriage. There is no reason to believe women in this study would be more or less motivated to remain in a relationship than other samples with women whose relationships range from dating to married.

In sum, the results of this study underscore two major points. First, conceptualization of psychological abuse should be expanded beyond the predominant approach which associates emotional or psychological abuse too closely with obviously dominating and controlling acts such as physical violence. Second, it is possible, indeed important, to differentiate obvious, overt, and subtle acts of psychological abuse. All three forms are harmful and can be measured.

NOTES

[1]Reporting the range of income would be misleading because determination of poverty status was based on federal tables comparing income and number of people in the household who depend on that income. During screening, the cutoff for income from work was 175%, hoping to obtain a sample living below 200% of poverty. Poverty status based on work alone ranged from 0% of the federal poverty level to 338% (M = 91.22%, Med = 93%). This was over 200% because women were also eligible if they received aid designed to alleviate poverty. Later it was discovered that official designations of poverty must include the cash value of public aid (e.g., food stamps, child care). When aid was included, calculations could be made for 817 women who knew the cash value of their aid and both partners' income from work if they were cohabiting. The cash value of aid is often not known by recipients for several reasons (e.g., food stamps are electronically updated monthly, child care is valued differently depending on the program providing it, with a rent subsidy women know what they pay rather than the value of their home). Using this procedure, poverty status ranged from 0% to 399% (M = 106.97%, Med = 106%). All but two women were receiving at least one type of aid. (The woman who was least poor at 399% of poverty received both Medicaid and food stamps.) In addition, women who had insufficient data with which to calculate poverty status all received aid. Thus, all women were very poor or among the most disadvantaged of the "working poor" which would likely cause them to rely on free public and private services.

[2]Space prohibits examination of the pattern of results for each racial/ethnic group. Although there were only minor group differences on some independent and dependent variables used in this study, different variables emerged as important in regression equations calculated within each group. However, the general pattern was the same, with subtle psychological abuse having more impact than overt psychological abuse or direct aggression. These similarities and differences will be reported in a later article.

REFERENCES

Acitelli, L. K., Douvan, E., & Veroff, J. (1989). *Perceptions of self and spouse during marital conflict.* Presented at the International Conference on Personal Relationships. University of Iowa, Iowa City.

Acitelli, L. K., Douvan, E., & Veroff, J. (1997). The changing influence of interpersonal perceptions on marital well-being among black and white couples. *Journal of Social and Personal Relationships, 14,* 291-304.

Arias, I., Lyons, C. M., & Street, A. E. (1997). Individual and marital consequences of victimization: Moderating effects of relationship efficacy and spouse support. *Journal of Family Violence, 12,* 193-210.

Babcock, J. C., Waltz, J., Jacobson, N. S., & Gottman, J. M. (1993). Power and violence: The relation between communication patterns, power discrepancies, and domestic violence. *Journal of Consulting and Clinical Psychology, 61,* 40-50.

Barnett, O., & Hamberger, L. (1992). The assessment of maritally violent men on the California Psychological Inventory. *Violence and Victims, 7,* 15-28.

Bergman, B., & Brismar, B. (1991). A 5-year follow-up study of 117 battered women. *American Journal of Public Health, 81,* 1486-1489.

Berry, W. D., & Feldman, S. (1985). *Multiple regression in practice.* Newbury Park, CA: Sage.

Brice-Baker, J. R. (1994). Domestic violence in African-American and African-Caribbean families. *Journal of Distress and the Homeless, 3,* 23-38.

Campbell, J. C. (1989). Women's response to sexual abuse in intimate relationships. *Health Care for Women International, 10,* 335-346.

Campbell, J. C., Miller, P., Cardwell, M. M., & Belknap, R. A. (1994). Relationship status of battered women over time. *Journal of Family Violence, 9,* 99-111.

Cascardi, M., Langhrinsen, J., & Vivian, D. (1992). Marital aggression: Impact, injury, and health correlates for husbands and wives. *Archives of Internal Medicine, 152,* 1178-84.

Cascardi, M., & O'Leary, K. D. (1992). Depressive symptomatology, self-esteem and self-blame in battered women. *Journal of Family Violence, 7,* 249-259.

Cascardi, M., & Vivian, D. (1995). Context for specific episodes of marital violence: Gender and severity of violence differences. *Journal of Family Violence, 10,* 265-293.

Cloven, D. H. & Roloff, M. E. (1991). *Sense-making activities and interpersonal conflict: Communicative cures for the mulling blues.* Western Journal of Speech Communication, 55, 134-158.

Cohen, S., Kamarck, T., & Mermelstein, R. (1983). A global measure of perceived stress. *Journal of Health and Social Behavior, 24,* 385-396.

Crohan, S. E., & Veroff, J. (1989). Dimensions of marital well-being among white and black newlyweds. *Journal of Marriage and the Family, 51,* 373-383.

Crowell, N. A., & Burgess, A. W. (1996). *Understanding violence against women.* Washington, DC: National Academy Press.

Derogatis, L. R., Lipman, R. S., & Covi, L. (1973). SCL-90: An outpatient psychiatric rating scale-preliminary report. *Psychopharmacology Bulletin, 9,* 13-28.

Dutton, M. A. (1992). Assessment and treatment of post-traumatic stress disorder among battered women. In D. W. Foy (Ed.), *Treating post-traumatic stress disorder: Cognitive behavioral strategies* (pp. 69-97). New York: Guilford Press.

Ellington, J. E., & Marshall, L. L. (1997). Gender role perceptions of women in abusive relationships. *Sex Roles, 36,* 349-369.

Follingstad, D. R., Rutledge, L. L., Berg, B. J., Hause, E. S., & Polek, D. S. (1990). The role of emotional abuse in physically abusive relationships. *Journal of Family Violence, 5,* 107-120.

Frieze, I. H., & McHugh, M. C. (1992). Power and influence strategies in violent and nonviolent marriages. *Psychology of Women Quarterly, 16,* 449-465.

Goldberg, D. P., & Hillier, V. F. (1979). A scaled version of the general health questionnaire. *Psychological Medicine, 9,* 139-145.

Gondolf, W. W., Fisher, E., & McFerron, J. R. (1990). The helpseeking behavior of battered women: An analysis of 6000 shelter interviews. In E. C. Viano (Ed.), *The victimology handbook: Research, treatment and public policy* (113-127). New York: Garland Publishing.

Hatchett, S., Veroff, J., & Douvan, E. (1995). Factors influencing marital stability among black and white couples. In B. Tucker & C. Mitchell-Kernan (Eds.), *The decline in marriages among African Americans: Causes, consequences and policy implications.* Newbury Park, CA: Sage.

Hays, R. D., Sherbourne, C. D., & Mazel, R. M. (1993). The RAND 36-item health survey 1.0. *Health Economics, 2,* 217-227.

Jacobson, N., Gottman, J., Gortner, E., Berns, S., & Shortt, J. (1996). Psychological factors in the longitudinal course of battering: When do the couples split up? When does the abuse decrease? *Violence and Victims, 11,* 371-392.

Jacobson, N., Gottman, J., Waltz, J., Rushe, R., Babcock, J., & Holtzworth-Munroe, A. (1994). Affect, verbal content and psychophysiology in the arguments of couples with a violent husband. *Journal of Clinical and Consulting Psychology, 62,* 982-988.

Kasian, M., & Painter, S. L. (1992). Frequency and severity of psychological abuse in a dating population. *Journal of Interpersonal Violence, 7,* 350-364.

Kelly, K. D., & DeKeseredy, W. S. (1994). Women's fear of crime and abuse in college and university dating relationships. *Violence and Victims, 9,* 17-30.

Kilpatrick, D. G., Best, C. L., Saunders, B. E., & Veronen, L. J. (1988). Rape in marriage and in dating relationships: How bad is it for mental health? *Annals of the New York Academy of Science, 528,* 335-344.

Kurz, D., & Stark, E. (1989). Not so benign neglect: The medical response to battering. In K. Yllo & M. Bograd (Eds.), *Feminist perspectives on wife abuse* (pp. 249-266). Newbury Park, CA: Sage.

Lloyd, S. A. (1996). Physical aggression, distress, and everyday marital interaction. In D. Cahn & S. Lloyd (Eds.), *Family violence from a communication perspective* (pp. 177-198). Newbury Park, CA: Sage.

Margolin, G., John, R. S., & Gleberman, L. (1988). Affective responses to conflictual discussions in violent and nonviolent couples. *Journal of Consulting and Clinical Psychology, 56,* 24-33.

Marshall, L. L. (1992a). Development of the Severity of Violence Against Women Scale. *Journal of Family Violence, 7,* 103-121.

Marshall, L. L. (1992b). The severity of Violence Against Men Scales. *Journal of Family Violence, 7,* 189-204.

Marshall, L. L. (1994). Physical and psychological abuse. In W. R. Cupach & B. H. Spitzberg (Eds.), *The dark side of interpersonal communication* (pp. 281-311). Hillsdale, NJ: Lawrence Erlbaum Associates.

Marshall, L. L. (1996). Psychological abuse of women: Six distinct clusters. *Journal of Family Violence, 11,* 369-399.

Marshall, L. L., & Guarnaccia, C. (1998). *Men's psychological-harm and abuse in relationships measure (MP-HARM): Overt and subtle psychological abuse.* Manuscript in preparation.

Marshall, L. L., & Rose, P. (1990). Gender, stress and violence in the adult relationships of a sample of college students. *Journal of Social and Personal Relationships, 4,* 299-316.

McCloskey, L. A. (1996). Socioeconomic and coercive power within the family. *Gender and Society, 10,* 449-463.

Mihalic, S., & Elliott, D. (1997). A social learning theory model of marital violence. *Journal of Family Violence, 12,* 21-47.

Murphy, C. M., & Cascardi, M. (1993). Psychological aggression and abuse in marriage. In R. L. Hamptom, T. P. Gullotta, S. R. Adams, E. H. Potter III, & R. P. Weissberg (Eds.), *Family violence: Prevention and treatment* (pp. 86-112). Newbury Park, CA: Sage.

Nolen-Hoeksema, S. (1987). Sex differences in unipolar depression: Evidence and theory. *Psychological Bulletin, 101,* 259-282.

O'Leary, K. D., & Jouriles, E. N. (1994). Psychological abuse between adult partners. In L. L'Abate (Ed.), *Handbook of developmental family psychology and psychopathology* (pp. 330-349). New York: John Wiley and Sons.

O'Leary, K. D., Malone, J., & Tyree, A. (1994). Physical aggression in early marriage: Prerelationship and relationship effects. *Journal of Consulting and Clinical Psychology, 62,* 594-602.

Pipes, R. B., & LeBov-Keeler, K. (1997). Psychological abuse among college women in exclusive heterosexual dating relationships. *Sex Roles, 36,* 585-603.

Riggs, D. S., Kilpatrick, D. G., & Resnick, H. C. (1992). Long-term psychological distress associated with marital rape and aggravated assault: A comparison to other crime victims. *Journal of Family Violence, 7,* 283-296.

Roberts, A. R. (1996). Battered women who kill: A comparative study of incarcerated participants with a community sample of battered women. *Journal of Family Violence, 11,* 291-304.

Rosenberg, M. (1965). *Society and the adolescent self-image.* Princeton, NJ: Princeton University Press.

Saunders, D. G. (1996). Feminist-cognitive-behavioral and process-psychodynamic treatment models for men who batter: Interaction of abuser traits and treatment models. *Violence and Victims, 11,* 393-414.

Shinn, M., Knickman, J. R., & Weitzman, B. C. (1991). Social relationships and vulnerability to becoming homeless. *American Psychologist, 46,* 1180-1188.

Sommers, E. K., & Check, J. V. P. (1987). An empirical investigation of the role of pornography in the verbal and physical abuse of women. *Violence and Victims, 2,* 189-209.

Stets, J. E. (1991) Psychological aggression in dating relationships: The role of interpersonal control. *Journal of Family Violence, 6,* 97-114.

Straus, M. A., Hamby, S. L., Boney-McCoy, S., & Sugarman, D. S. (1996). The revised Conflict Tactics Scale (CTS2): Development and preliminary psychometric data. *Journal of Family Violence, 17,* 283-316.

Stuart, E. P., & Campbell, J. C. (1989). Assessment of patterns of dangerousness with battered women. *Issues in Mental Health Nursing, 10,* 245-260.

Trope, Y., & Liberman, A. (1996). Social hypothesis testing: Cognitive and motivational mechanisms. In E. T. Higgins & A. W. Kruglanski (Eds.), *Social psychology handbook of basic principles* (pp. 239-270). NY: Guilford Press.

Vitanza, S., Vogel, L. C. M., & Marshall, L. L. (1995). Distress and symptoms of posttraumatic stress disorder in abused women. *Violence and Victims, 10,* 23-34.

Vivian, D., & Malone, J. (1997). Couples at risk for husband-to-wife violence: Screening potential of marital assessment inventories. *Violence and Victims, 12,* 1-19.

Wood, D., Valdez, B., Hayashi, T., & Shen, A. (1990). Homeless and housed families in Los Angeles. *American Journal of Public Health, 80,* 1049-1052.

Zawitz, M. W. (1994). *Violence between intimates.* Bureau of Justice Statistics, report #NCJ149259 available from BJS, P. O. Box 179, Annapolis Junction, MD 20701-0179.

Chapter 10

Court-Involved Battered Women's Responses to Violence: The Role of Psychological, Physical, and Sexual Abuse

Mary Ann Dutton, Lisa A. Goodman, and Lauren Bennett

omestic violence research has continued to expand over the past two decades. Yet only recently has research begun to examine systematically the role of psychological abuse in the context of physically violent relationships. While the severity of physical violence is an important element of battered women's experience, it is critical to understand the entire configuration of coercive control tactics (Stark, 1995). Coercive control can be accomplished through psychological abuse, maintaining control achieved through physical means (Ganley, 1989).

Psychological abuse, along with physical abuse, sexual abuse, and abuse to property and pets (Ascione, 1998) are major dimensions of intimate partner violence (Ganley, 1989). More than half of a community sample of physically abused battered women (Follingstad, Rutledge, Berg, Hause, & Polek, 1990) reported a high frequency (i.e., once a week or more) of three types of emotional abuse: restriction, batterer jealousy, and ridicule. Higher levels of psychological abuse have been reported in physically abusive than in either dissatisfied, but nonabusive, or satisfied relationships (Carbone, 1996; Tolman, 1999). Furthermore, O'Leary and his colleagues (O'Leary, Malone, & Tyree, 1994) have shown that psychological abuse significantly predicts the development of physical abuse in marital relationships.

Few studies to date have focused on battered women in the justice system. While most studies have included shelter or community samples, we know far less about women who seek legal remedies—either civil or criminal. The justice system is a critical point of contact and intervention for some battered women yet, in two multistate studies, between 25% and 56% of women did not obtain permanent civil protection orders following the issuance of a temporary order (Keilitz, Hannaford, & Efkeman, 1997), mostly because the batterer stopped bothering her. Prosecutors have developed "no drop" policies and other responses to the problem of uncooperative victims in the criminal prosecution of domestic violence cases (Rebovich, 1996). We know little about what specific factors contribute to women's decisions not to use court resources.

The aim of this study was to investigate the relative role of psychological, physical, and sexual intimate partner abuse among predominately African American women involved in the criminal justice system in shaping strategic and traumatic stress responses to intimate partner violence.

Predicting Women's Strategic Responses to Violence

Strategic responses are defined as helpseeking and other types of behaviors battered women employ to protect themselves and their children from domestic violence (Dutton, 1993). Research has shown that battered women are active in their help-seeking effort (Gondolf & Fisher, 1988; Hutchinson & Ahirschel, 1998). Some previous research has examined the relationship between abuse characteristics and women's strategic responses to violence. A study of shelter women (Gondolf & Fisher, 1988) found that the severity of wife abuse (defined by physical abuse, verbal abuse, and injury) per se, was not significantly associated with an increase in number of help-seeking efforts. However, increased help-seeking was observed in the context of batterers' antisocial behavior or negative behavior toward the victim following the abuse, suggesting that battered women may be responding to men they view as generally dangerous (Gondolf & Fisher, 1988). A study involving a nationally representative sample (Kantor & Straus, 1990) found that police were involved in cases of severe violence between couples four times more often than in cases of minor violence, but who made the calls to police was not specifically examined. A recent study of urban, predominately African American women found that greater severity of physical violence, greater tangible support (e.g., to borrow money, offer transportation), and having children in common with the batterer, predicted battered women's cooperation with criminal prosecution (Goodman, Bennett, & Dutton, in press).

Only a few studies have included physical, psychological, and sexual components of the intimate partner violence in their study of women's help-seeking. One such study (Marshall, 1996), found psychological abuse, threats, violent acts, and sexual aggression predicted whether women from a community sample had ever had contact with any help-seeking source as well as the number of sources contacted. Contact with the court was predicted by threats of violence and psychological abuse, while contact with police was predicted by threats of violence, violent acts, and psychological abuse. Still, we know little about what predicts how women use the help-seeking resources once they have contact with them.

A recent study (Dutton et al., 1999), using the same sample of predominately African American battered women in the court system as in the present study, found that women's cooperation with prosecution was best predicted by whether the woman had children in common with the batterer, severity of total violence (defined by physical assault, violence, and sexual abuse), tangible support, and lower scores reflecting problems with alcohol. However, psychological abuse was not examined in these comparisons.

Another important legal remedy for battered women is the civil protection order, that is, a civil order issued by a judge with specific remedies attached. A recent study involving three cities (Keilitz et al., 1997) found these remedies included an order for the batterer not to abuse the victim (e.g., assault, threaten) (92%), to have no contact with the victim (55%), to stay away from the victim's home or place of work (80%), to vacate the home (32%), and to attend batterer counseling (25%). These orders often have provisions concerning the children as well, including custody granted to the petitioner/victim (80%), order to pay child support (37%), and denial of visitation (10%). Thus, the civil protection order can provide for a wide array of remedies for the domestic violence victim, although enforcement of the civil protection order is a key issue. However, there has been scant research examining predictors of women's follow-through with obtaining permanent civil protection orders once having filed a petition requesting one. One study of predominately White participants (Gondolf, McWilliams, Hart, & Stuehling, 1994) found in a review of court records that being married was the only background variable related to whether the women obtained the protective order. Another study (Harrell, Smith, & Newmark, 1993) reported that African American, younger women, and women who had not given a copy of the temporary order to police were less likely to return to the court for the final civil protection order hearing. Variables in that study not related to returning to court were the woman's educational level, employment status, whether she had children, whether she lived with the abusive partner, length of relationship, duration of abuse, and severity of incident that led to the temporary order. However, a recent study involving predominately White, married battered women (Fischer, Campbell, & Rappaport, in press) found that women reporting greater severity and duration of abuse, as well as the perception that abuse was escalating, were more likely to return to court. Notably, none of these studies included predominately African American women. Further, none included measures of psychological—as well as physical—abuse.

Leaving the abusive relationship is another strategic response to violence, one which has been studied more extensively. Abuse variables have been linked to battered women's remaining in or leaving an abusive relationship. Several studies have found that women who leave their abusive partners report more severe violence (for a review see Strube, 1988). Consistent with these findings, a study of sheltered battered women (Rusbult & Martz, 1995) found that higher levels of commitment, which, in turn, were associated with less severe abuse, were related to returning to an abusive partner. Most studies which have addressed the link between abuse characteristics and leaving have focused on physical—but not psychological—abuse. A recent exception is a study of married couples (Jacobson, Gottman, Gortner, Berns, & Shortt, 1996) which found that women who were separated reported higher levels of husband emotional abuse (including isolation and degradation) at Time 1 than women still in the relationship 2 years later. Further, husband emotional abuse was a stronger predictor of separation/divorce than physical violence (Gortner, Jacobson, Berns, & Gottman, 1997).

In sum, most research on battered women's strategic response to violence has not included measures of both psychological and physical abuse. Further, most studies to date have included samples of predominately White women, thus we know little about the strategic responses by women in other ethnic groups. The present study aims to address these shortcomings.

Predicting Traumatic Stress Effects of Violence

Traumatic stress effects of violence and other traumatic experiences have been widely studied (van der Kolk, McFarlane, & Weisaeth, 1996; Wilson & Raphael, 1993) across various populations, such as combat veterans, victims of natural disaster, child abuse, and victims of violent assault. A recent meta-analysis (Weaver & Clum, 1995) examined the impact of violence dimensions on psychological outcomes and concluded that the study results demonstrated only a moderate relationship between objective measures of violence (e.g., amount of force, injury, use of a weapon) and psychological distress. Interestingly, however, subjective factors (e.g., general appraisal, life threat, self-blame, perceived controllability) were more strongly associated with psychological distress. The impact of different dimensions of intimate partner abuse on the psychological functioning has yet to be adequately studied—specifically the relative effects of physical, psychological, and sexual abuse.

Studies of domestic violence have found that greater severity of partner violence reported by battered women has been associated with more serious psychological effects (Follingstad, Brenan, Hause, Polek, & Rutledge, 1991), including depression (Campbell, Kub, Belknap, & Templin, 1997; Cascardi & O'Leary, 1992; Tuel & Russell, 1998), suicide (Kaslow et al., 1998), and posttraumatic stress disorder (Houskamp & Foy, 1991; Kemp, Green, Horowitz, & Rawlins, 1995). However, only a few studies have included measures of both physical and psychological abuse as predictors of psychological distress. An early study of psychological abuse (Follingstad et al., 1990) found that 72% of a community sample of physically battered women reported the impact of the psychological abuse to be worse than the impact of physical abuse. Another study (Campbell et al., 1997) found nonphysical abuse to be significantly correlated with depression, but multivariate analyses failed to find a significant effect. A recent study of African American women (Kaslow et al., 1998) found that even after the effects of child maltreatment were controlled for, nonphysical, but not physical, partner abuse was significantly related to having attempted suicide. The present study was designed to begin to fill a significant gap in the existing literature (Campbell & Lewandowski, 1997) concerning the differential effects of physical, sexual, and emotional victimization on battered women's strategic responses and mental health.

METHOD

Participants

One hundred forty-nine women who sought assistance from a domestic violence intake center located in the court were recruited for participation in the study. Women sought help from the court because they were interested in obtaining a civil protection order and/or participating in the criminal prosecution against a current or former abusive partner (referred to an index partner). Of the 149 participants, 75 (50%) both wanted a protection order and had a criminal case pending against their abusive partner; 16 (11%) had not filed a protection order but were involved in a criminal case against their partner, and 58 (39%) wanted a protection order but were not involved in the criminal justice system at the time of the study. Participants were predominately African American (91%) with 2.5%, Anglo; 1.9%, Latina; 1.2%, Asian American; and 3.1%, Other. The mean age of the sample was 30 years, with a range of 18 to 58 years. Most often, the abusive partner was an ex-boyfriend (47.5%) or current boyfriend (28.4%); the rest were married to (18.5%) or divorced or separated from (5.5%) an abusive partner. The average length of relationship was 4.42 years (range: 1 month to 35 years). Half of the participants had been married less than 3 years. Approximately one-third of the sample (32.5%) was coresiding with the abusive partner at the time of recruitment. Only 13.8% of women reported being financially dependent on the batterer. Almost half (46%) were employed; most of these were employed full time (83.8%). Most women had at least one child (74.1%), and half (50%) had a child in common with their abusive partner.

Measures

Background Questionnaire. An initial paper-and-pencil questionnaire was administered during the court intake process and was used to elicit information concerning age, ethnicity, housing status, current relationship status, length of relationship, number of dependent children, children in common with the batterer, employment status, economic dependence on batterer. A follow-up questionnaire was administered by phone between 2–4 weeks following the filing of the petition for participants who had filed a civil protection order and again at 12 weeks for those for whom there was a criminal case involving their abusive partner. Only data from the 12-week follow-up contact are reported here.

Predictor Variables. Three subscales of the *Revised Conflict Tactics Scale* (CTS-2)-Form A (Straus, Hamby, Boney-McCoy, & Sugarman, 1995) were administered at intake to assess physical assault (CTS2-P; 12 items), injury (CTS2-I; 6 items), and sexual coercion (CTS2-S; 7 items). Participants made frequency ratings (range = 1 or "never or not in the past year" to 6 or "more than 20 times in the past year") which were summed to produce an index of severity of violence by the index partner over the last year. Cronbach alpha coefficients for the participants in this study were .76 for Injury, .82 for Sexual Coercion, and .91 for Physical Assault.

The *Psychological Maltreatment of Women Inventory* (PMWI) (Tolman, 1989) was administered at intake to assess severity of psychological abuse. The PMWI consists of two factor-analytically derived subscales: dominance/isolation (PMWI-D/I) and emotional/verbal (PMWI-E/V). Both subscales of the PMWI-Short Form scores have been found to correlate highly with the nonphysical subscale of the Index of Spouse Abuse (Hudson & McIntosh, 1981), another commonly used scale for measuring psychological abuse. Further, scores on the PMWI have been found to differentiate women in three types of relationships: physically abusive, dissatisfied but not physically abusive, and satisfied (Carbone, 1996; Tolman, 1999). Reliability coefficients for the present sample were .85 for emotional/verbal (PMWI-E/V) and .82 for dominance/isolation (PMWI-D/I).

Strategic Response Outcome Variables. Information concerning participants' prior use of specific strategies to response to domestic violence was obtained in the initial self-report questionnaire administered at intake. These variables included whether the participant had previously called the police and whether she had previously left the abusive relationship. Based on a median split, information about whether the participant had previously left the abusive partner was categorized as 0–1 times vs. twice or more times.

Current coping strategies included a measure of cooperation with criminal prosecution and follow-through with civil protection orders. Information on cooperation with prosecution was obtained from prosecutors for each case on the first scheduled trial date, regardless of the status of the case at that time. The first trial date was chosen because it occurs at approximately the same point in time (12 weeks after intake) in every case, and it is a time when the prosecutor typically makes contact with the victim. On a sticker attached to the front of each victim's prosecution file, the prosecutor indicated whether the victim was "cooperative" with the prosecution at that point. Cooperation was defined as the victim's willingness to come to court and to testify for the prosecution, if necessary. In those cases ($n = 18$) where the prosecutor failed to provide a cooperation rating, information from the 3-month follow-up phone call was used instead. In this case, "cooperation" was defined as participant's report of having appeared in court on the first trial date or having been willing to do so, if requested. If participants reported that they were generally committed to cooperating with prosecutors but did not appear in court on the appropriate day for whatever reason, they were rated as uncooperative. In those cases where both prosecutor and interviewer ratings were available ($n = 37$), the two ratings were perfectly correlated.

Follow-through with civil protection orders was determined from information obtained in the court jacket. "Follow-through" was defined as showing up in court to go forward with the petition at the permanent hearing 2 weeks after intake. "Not following through" was defined as either not showing up in court or showing up for the purpose of asking the court to withdraw the petition.

Traumatic Stress Outcome Variables. The *Center for Epidemiological Studies—Depression Scale* (CES-D) (Radloff, 1977) was administered at intake to assess depression. Participants reported the number of times they had experienced each of 20 depressive symptoms over the week prior to the interview. The total score reflects severity of depression. This scale has been used extensively with community samples of low-income women (Belle, 1982; Goodman, 1991). Previous research with community and psychiatric inpatient samples (Radloff, 1977) have shown a cutoff score of 16 as indicative of clinical depression. Cronbach's alpha for this sample was .90.

The Stanford Acute Stress Reaction Questionnaire (SASRQ; Spiegel, Koopman, Classen, & Cardena,) was administered at intake to assess symptoms of acute stress disorder. The 30-item measure is designed to assess DSM-IV criteria for Acute Stress Disorder (Cardena, 1996). Scores reflecting frequency ranged from 0–150. The alpha reliability coefficient for the current sample was .96.

The revised DSM-IV version of the 17-item Posttraumatic Stress Disorder Symptom Scale-Self-Report (PSS-SR; Foa, Riggs, Dancu, & Rothbaum, 1993) was administered during the 12-week follow-up phone contact to assess symptoms of PTSD. A sum score (0–51) reflecting severity was used. The Cronbach alpha reliability coefficient was .92 for the current sample. The PSS-SR was administered at the follow-up phone interview because DSM-IV criteria require at least 1 month following the stressor event for symptoms to be considered indicative of PTSD. Thus, PTSD measures were obtained only for those women for whom there was a criminal case pending against an abusive partner, that is, on 61% of the sample. In a validity study using the SCID (Foa et al., 1993), sensitivity was 62% and specificity was 100%. Positive prediction power was 100% and negative predictive power was 82%.

Procedure

Women who sought help at a domestic violence intake center located within a coordinated domestic violence court project were recruited for participation in the study. Women were recruited for the study immediately after meeting with a victim advocate. After participants signed a consent form giving permission to participate in the study, including the two follow-up phone contacts, they completed a set of questionnaires in a semiprivate area of the courthouse. Questionnaires required approximately 45 to 60 minutes to complete. Participants were paid $10 for their participation. Follow-up phone calls were made 3–4 weeks following the initial interview for women who filed a petition for the civil protection order (data from this follow-up contact are not included in this study) and again at 12 weeks for women where there had been a criminal case filed against their abusive partner.

Data Analysis

Linear (continuous outcome variables) and logistic (dichotomous outcome variables) regression analyses were used to determine the relative predictive value of psychological, physical, and sexual abuse variables. Univariate analyses were first conducted in order to examine the unique relationship between each predictor and outcome. Then multivariate analyses were performed to determine the predictive value of each variable taking into account the others. In the case of logistic regression, odds ratios were calculated for a one standard deviation change in the predictor variable.

RESULTS

Preliminary Analyses

All correlations among the physical, sexual, and psychological abuse (i.e., predictor) variables were significant and ranged from .31 to 80. As indicated in Table 1, the pattern of correlations suggests that the subscales of the CTS2 and PMWI, as measures of physical assault, injury, sexual abuse, and psychological abuse, tap separate components of the domestic violence experience, with the exception of the expected overlap between physical assault and injury. Table 2 indicates the means and standard deviations for the predictor variables as well as the percentage of participants who reported "severe" abuse as measured by the CTS2 (Straus et al., 1995). The levels of dominance/isolation (PMWI-D/I) (M = 21.96) and emotional/verbal (PMWI-E/V) (M = 25.04) psychological abuse are remarkably comparable to scores for Tolman's (1999) sample of service-seeking battered women of 20.3 and 25.6, respectively.

Table 1. Correlations Between Abuse Variables

	CTS2-P	CTS2-I	CTS2-S	PMWI D/I	PMWI E/V
CTS2 - Physical	–	.80***	.48***	.31***	.34***
CTS2 - Injury		–	.55***	.33***	.32***
CTS2 - Sexual			–	.32***	.32***
PMWI - D/I				–	.65***

Note. CTS2-P = Physical Assault, CTS2-I = Injury, CTS2-S = Sexual Coercion subscales of the Revised Conflict Tactics Scale. PMWI-D/I = Dominance / Isolation, PMWI-E/V = Emotional / Verbal subscales of the Psychological Maltreatment of Women Inventory. ***$p \leq .001$.

Table 2. Means and Standard Deviations for Abuse Measures ($n = 164$)

Abuse Measure	Possible Range	Mean	Standard Deviation
CTS2 - Total	25-150	30.67	26.53
CTS2 - Injury	6-36	5.97	6.15
CTS2 - Physical	12-72	19.36	15.96
CTS2 - Sexual	7-42	5.29	8.19
PMWI - Total	14-70	47.41	13.69
PMWI - Dominance	7-35	21.96	7.53
PMWI - Emotional	7-35	25.04	7.51

Note. CTS2-P = Physical Assault, CTS2-I = Injury, CTS2-S = Sexual Coercion subscales of the Revised Conflict Tactics Scale. PMWI - D/I = Dominance / Isolation, PMWI-E/V = Emotional / Verbal subscales of the Psychological Maltreatment of Women Inventory.

Predicting Use of Prior and Current Strategic Responses

Regarding previous responses to domestic violence, 72% of participants had previously called the police and 84% had made two or more previous attempts to leave the relationship with the index abusive partner. Participants' average number of prior attempts to leave was 2.7 times. Among those who had ever left, the mean number of times leaving the abusive relationship was 3.3. Demographic variables, including age, marital status with the abusive partner about whom she had contacted with the court, and length of relationship, were not significantly correlated with any of the strategic response variables.

Among participants for whom there was a current criminal case pending against their abusive partner ($n = 92$ or 56% of the sample), 48% were rated by prosecutors 3 months later as fully cooperative as a victim/witness in the criminal case. Thirty-six percent of the participants who had filed for a civil protection order (89% of the sample) followed through to obtain a permanent order which was issued at a final

Table 3. Univariate Logistic Regression of Abuse Variables on Participants' Prior and Current Strategic Responses to Intimate Partner Violence

Predictor Variables	B	*SE*	Wald	Odds Ratio[a]
Prior Attempts to Leave the Abusive Relationship (0-1 vs. 2 or more)				
CTS2 - Physical	.03	.01	4.82*	1.67
CTS2 - Injury	.10	.04	4.84*	1.82
CTS2 - Sexual	.05	.05	1.05	1.39
PMWI - D/I	.05	.04	1.64	1.46
PMWI - E/V	.02	.04	.32	1.19
Prior Call(s) to Police (Yes/No)				
CTS2 - Physical	-.05	.01	11.23***	2.22
CTS2 - Injury	-.17	.05	12.59***	2.84
CTS2 - Sexual	-.06	.03	3.86*	1.63
PMWI - D/I	-.09	.02	11.82***	1.97
PMWI - E/V	-.07	.02	7.78**	1.69
Current Cooperation With Criminal Prosecution (Yes/No)				
CTS2 - Physical	-.03	.01	5.46*	1.69
CTS2 - Injury	-.09	.04	4.69*	1.74
CTS2 - Sexual	-.01	.02	.38	1.13
PMWI - D/I	-.07	.03	4.94*	1.69
PMWI - E/V	-.04	.03	2.25	1.35
Current Follow-Through With Civil Protection Order (Yes/No)				
CTS2 - Physical	.01	.01	.53	1.14
CTS2 - Injury	.01	.03	.06	1.04
CTS2 - Sexual	-.01	.02	.36	1.11
PMWI - D/I	-.04	.02	3.63	1.35
PMWI - E/V	-.04	.02	3.30	1.35

Note. CTS2-P = Physical Assault, CTS2-I = Injury, and CTS2-S = Sexual Coercion subscales of the Revised Conflict Tactics Scale (CTS2). PMWI-D/I = Dominance / Isolation and PMWI-E/V = Emotional / Verbal subscales of the Psychological Maltreatment of Women Inventory (PMWI).
[a]Odds ratios are calculated for a 1 SD change in the predictor variables.
*$p \leq .05$, **$p \leq .01$, ***$p \leq .001$.

hearing either by consent (75% of those who received an order) or after a hearing (25%). In some cases, the protection order hearing was continued and the final hearing was scheduled more than 2 weeks subsequent to the initial petition. Follow-through was determined by the final disposition at whatever point it occurred.

There was a significant positive correlation in those cases which involved both a petition for a civil protection order and a pending criminal case ($n = 75$) between following through with the civil protection order and cooperating with criminal prosecution ($r = .35$, $p \leq .001$). Women who returned to obtain the permanent civil protection order were more likely to cooperate with criminal prosecution.

Table 4. Multivariate Logistic Regression of Abuse Variables on Participants' Prior and Current Strategic Responses to Intimate Partner Violence

Predictor Variable	B	SE	Wald	Odds Ratio[a]
Attempts to Leave the Abusive Relationship[b]				
CTS2 - Injury	.10	.04	4.84*	1.81
Prior Call(s) to Police[c]				
CTS2 - Injury	-.15	.05	9.13**	2.54
PMWI - D/I	-.07	.03	6.22**	1.65
Cooperation With Criminal Prosecution[d]				
CTS2 - Physical	-.03	.01	5.46*	1.69

Note. CTS2-P = Physical Assault and CTS2-I = Injury subscales of the Revised Conflict Tactics Scale (CTS2). PMWI-D/I = Dominance / Isolation subscale of the Psychological Maltreatment of Women Inventory (PMWI).
[a]Odds ratios are calculated for 1 S.D. change in the predictor variables.
[b]Hosmer-Lemeshow (C) Chi-square goodness-of-fit = 7.4, $p < .50$,
Correct classification = 57.3%
[c]Hosmer-Lemeshow (C) Chi-square goodness-of-fit = 8.6, $p < .37$,
Correct classification = 72.6%
[d]Hosmer-Lemeshow (C) Chi-square goodness-of-fit = 10.7, $p < .22$,
Correct classification = 59.8%.
*$p = .05$, **$p = .01$, ***$p = .001$.

Logistic regression analyses were conducted to predict participants' use of both previous and current strategies in response to domestic violence from the index partner. Previously used strategies included whether the victim ever left the abusive partner or previously called the police. Current strategies included whether the victim cooperated with criminal prosecution against the abusive partner and whether she followed through with the civil protection order petition.

Number of Prior Attempts to Leave Relationship. Participants were divided into two groups based on number of times they had previously left the abusive partner. The median split resulted in one group defined as 0-1 times and the other defined as leaving twice or more times. At the univariate level, only injury and physical assault predicted having left the abusive partner. However, only level of injury (CTS2-I) during the past year was significant at the multivariate level, indicating that a one standard deviation increase in injury score was associated with a 1.8 greater chance of having previously left the abusive relationship (twice or more times).

Previous Calls to Police. Univariate analyses revealed that all five abuse variables significantly predicted whether participants had previously called the police. However, only injury (CTS2-I) and dominance/isolation (PMWI-D/I) were

**Table 5. Univariate Linear Regression of Abuse Variables
on Participants' Traumatic Stress Responses**

Predictor Variables	B	SE	t	Adj. R²
Current Depression (CES-D) - Severity Level				
CTS2 - Physical	.25	.06	3.80***	.08
CTS2 - Injury	.59	.17	3.52***	.06
CTS2 - Sexual	.42	.13	3.34***	.06
PMWI - D/I	.81	.13	6.28***	.19
PMWI - E/V	.87	.13	6.87***	.22
Acute Stress (ASD) - Severity Level				
CTS2 - Physical	.91	.18	4.96***	.13
CTS2 - Injury	2.34	.48	4.93***	.12
CTS2 - Sexual	1.49	.36	4.08***	.09
PMWI - D/I	2.79	.35	7.88***	.27
PMWI - E/V	2.75	.36	7.71***	.26
Posttraumatic Stress Disorder (PTSD) - Severity Level				
CTS2 - Physical	.17	.05	3.11**	.09
CTS2 - Injury	.53	.14	3.87***	.13
CTS2 - Sexual	.25	.11	2.31*	.05
PMWI - D/I	.40	.11	3.55***	.11
PMWI - E/V	.54	.11	5.01***	.21

Note. CTS2-P = Physical Assault, CTS2-I = Injury, and CTS2-S = Sexual Coercion subscales of the Revised Conflict Tactics Scale (CTS2).
PMWI-D/I = Dominance / Isolation and PMWI-E/V = Emotional / Verbal subscales of the Psychological Maltreatment of Women Inventory (PMWI).
$*p \le .05$, $**p \le .01$, $***p \le .001$.

retained in the multivariate logistic regression, indicating that for every *SD* increase in injury level (CTS2-I) participants were more than 2.5 times more likely to have previously called the police. Likewise, one *SD* increase in dominance/isolation (PMWI-D/I) was associated with a 1.65 times greater likelihood of having previously called the police.

Current Cooperation With Criminal Prosecution. Cooperation with criminal prosecution was significantly predicted at the univariate level by level of physical assault (CTS2-P), injury (CTS2-I), and dominance/isolation (PMWI-D/I), but only level of physical assault (CTS2-P) was significant at the multivariate level. One SD increase in level of physical assault was associated with a 1.69 times increase in the likelihood of cooperating with criminal prosecution.

Current Follow-Through With Civil Protection Orders. None of the predictor variables significantly predicted at the univariate level whether participants returned to the court to obtain a permanent (1-year) protection order; thus, no multivariate analyses were conducted.

**Table 6. Multivariate Linear Regression of Abuse Variables
on Participants' Traumatic Stress Responses**

Predictor Variables	B	SE	t	Cum. Adj. R^2
Current Depression (Severity Level)				
PMWI - E/V	.62	.17	3.64***	.24
PMWI - D/I	.44	.17	2.59**	.27
Acute Stress (Severity Level)				
PMWI - D/I	1.61	.46	3.46***	.30
PMWI - E/V	1.54	.46	3.31***	.35
CTS2 - Injury	1.09	.44	2.48**	.37
Posttraumatic Stress Disorder (Severity Level)				
PMWI - E/V	.69	.20	3.45***	.37
CTS2 - Injury	.62	.27	2.26*	.42

Note. CTS2-I = Injury subscale of the Conflict Tactics Scale (CTS2). PMWI-D/I = Dominance / Isolation and PMWI-E/V = Emotional / Verbal subscales of the Psychological Maltreatment of Women Inventory (PMWI). $*p \leq .05$, $**p \leq .01$, $***p \leq .001$.

Predicting Traumatic Stress Responses

The mean score for depression (CES-D) was 27.38 ($SD = 13.7$). Seventy-four percent of the women had CES-D scores above the clinical cutoff of 16 (Radloff, 1977). The mean score for acute stress (SASRQ) was 63.47 ($SD = 39.2$) and for posttraumatic stress disorder symptoms (PSS-SR) was 14.14 ($SD = 8.61$). DSM-IV criteria for posttraumatic stress disorder (PTSD) were met by 39.6% ($n = 48$) of participants and DSM-IV criteria for acute stress disorder (ASD) were met by 40.1% ($n = 157$) of participants.

Depression. Univariate analyses revealed that all abuse variables—psychological, physical, and sexual abuse, and injury—predicted level of current depression. The final multivariate predictive model retained the two psychological abusive variables (PMWI-D/I, PMWI-E/V) only, which together explained 27% of the variance in severity of depression.

Acute Stress. Similarly, univariate analyses showed that all abuse variables predicted level of acute stress symptoms. The final multivariate predictive model included both psychological abuse variables (PMWI-D/I, PMWI-E/V) and level of injury (CTS2-I). Together, these variables explained 37% of the variance in level of acute stress.

PTSD. Finally, univariate analyses again revealed that all abuse variables predicted level of PTSD symptoms at follow-up. The final multivariate predictive model retained emotional/verbal abuse (PMWI-E/V) and level of injury (CTS2-I). Cumulatively, these two variables explained 23% of the variance in level of PTSD symptoms.

DISCUSSION

The relatively modest, albeit significant, correlations found between measures of physical (CTS-P, CTS-I, and CTS-S) and psychological (PMWI-D/I, PMWI-E/V) abuse provide empirical support for the notion that these variables measure different aspects of the abuse experience and, thus, for the importance of including measures of psychological abuse—not physical abuse alone—in future research on domestic violence. The correlations between psychological and physical abuse were considerably lower than in other reported research (Kaslow et al., 1998) which involved African American women from a health care setting and using different measures. This suggests the need for continued study of the overlap between different components of intimate partner violence.

Strategic Responses to Intimate Partner Violence

Results show that *prior attempts to leave the abusive relationship* were predicted by physical assault and injury, but not by sexual or psychological abuse even when considering the variables one at a time. Due to the high correlation between physical assault and injury, it is not surprising that when considered together only more severe injury predicted prior attempt to leave the relationship. These results are similar to findings from another group of researchers (Marshall, 1996) who also reported that physical, but not psychological, abuse predicted number of times battered women left an abusive partner. Interestingly, however, is that they found physical abuse, but not psychological abuse, predicted leaving only for some subgroups of battered women in the study, but the opposite results were observed for other subgroups of abused women. Further, the present results are inconsistent with findings by Gortner and colleagues (1997) that a husband's emotional state was a stronger predictor of marital dissolution than was physical violence. However, Gortner and associates' (1997) study did not specifically report results concerning women's role in leaving the relationship—only whether the relationship had been dissolved by either or both parties. At this point, understanding the role of psychological, compared to physical, abuse in battered women's decisions to leave abusive relationships requires further analysis of the context in which the abuse occurs (Dutton, 1996).

   Whether participants had ever *previously called the police* was found to be more likely when each of five types of physical and psychological abuse was rated as more serious. When each variable was considered taking into account each of the others, only more severe injury and greater dominance/isolation were found to offer significant and independent contributions to predicting prior calls to police. In the present study, injury was the more powerful predictor of police calls. For example, a woman whose report of injury was one standard deviation above the mean for the sample, was more than $2^{1}/_{2}$ times more likely to have called the police than a woman whose report of injury was at the mean for the group. These results are consistent with those found in the National Family Violence Re-Survey (Kantor & Straus, 1990) which reported that police were four times more likely to be involved when there had been severe, compared to minor, violence. However, these researchers did not examine the role of psychological factors in police calls. Like the present study, however, Marshall and associates (1996) also found that both physical and psychological abuse contributed to police calls. The present results support earlier findings that greater severity of violence leads to greater help-seeking efforts (Gondolf & Fisher, 1988) insofar as their measure of abuse included both verbal and physical abuse. It is noteworthy that even after the effects of injury were accounted for, greater dominance/isolation still increased the odds of calls to police by 50%. These data that women seek help from police more, not less, often when their abusive partner has made more efforts to dominate and isolate them support the notion that battered women make active efforts to resist the coercive control tactics—both physical and nonphysical—of their partners.

Physical abuse played a significant role in predicting *current cooperation with criminal prosecution.* Moreover, controlling for the influence of each of the other types of abuse, only physical assault contributed to predicting cooperation with current criminal prosecution. Although greater dominance/isolation and injury were predictive of cooperation when considered separately, these effects were not retained in the full model when the effects of physical violence were accounted for. When considering that the criminal justice code is based largely on the commission of overt acts, these results are not surprising. Perhaps the more serious the acts of physical violence and the more serious the criminal offense, the more likely battered women are to receive encouragement to cooperate with criminal prosecution.

None of the abuse variables explained either participants' prior use or current follow-through with civil protection orders. Previous findings which suggest that battered women often experience long histories of abuse prior to filing a civil protection order petition (Keilitz et al., 1997), along with the current results, indicate that there is much more to be understood about women's use of the court system in relation to civil protection orders.

Taken together, these results support the conclusion that different abuse configurations contribute differentially to battered women's strategic responses to abuse. Particularly interesting is the finding that physical abuse is central to predicting battered women's use of legal remedies as well as their decisions to leave the abusive relationship. The extent to which women in this study had begun to engage the help of the legal system (i.e., call police, criminal prosecution) as well as to leave the abusive relationship, was largely determined by greater severity of physical acts of violence (i.e., physical assault) and their physical consequences (i.e., injury). Recent developments in looking at battered women's stages of change (Brown, 1997), that is, a process by which women move from failing to recognize the abuse as a problem to active attempts to deal with it to maintaining safety, may be helpful in placing the findings of this and similar research in context. Accordingly, we need further research which examines predictors of different types of strategies within the same study—in addition to use of the legal system and leaving the abusive relationship.

Traumatic Stress Responses to Intimate Partner Violence

At the univariate level, all three types of traumatic response (e.g., depression, acute stress, and posttraumatic stress disorder symptoms) were associated with each of the five types of abuse, although, almost without exception, psychological abuse explained more variance than did physical abuse. Psychological abuse also played a more significant role when the variables were considered in context of each other, although severity of injury increased prediction of both acute and posttraumatic stress, but not depression.

With regard to both acute and posttraumatic stress disorder symptoms, the more serious the physical assault, injury, and sexual abuse—when considered separately—the more severe the symptoms. Generally, however, these physical abuse dimensions contributed only small portions of variance in explaining stress disorder symptoms. Surprisingly, measures of psychological abuse contributed larger portions of variance than did measures of physical abuse. When considered together, the most parsimonious set of predictors of acute stress disorder were dominance/isolation psychological abuse, emotional/verbal psychological abuse, and injury, with injury contributing only a small portion of additional variance. Predictors of posttraumatic stress disorder symptoms were similar in that most of the variance was explained by emotional/verbal psychological abuse with a small portion of variance added by injury. These data suggest that, in the context of physical assault (i.e., all participants had been physically assaulted), it is the psychological abuse experience that is more determinative of stress disorder symptoms. These findings are consistent with those of others (Kemp et al., 1995) who found verbal, as well as physical, abuse to be associated with PTSD.

Results concerning the prediction of depression in battered women are interesting in comparison to recent data of other researchers (cf. Campbell et al., 1997) who found both physical and nonphysical abuse to be correlated with battered women's depression. In the present study, each of the physical abuse dimensions (i.e., physical assault, injury, sexual coercion), taken separately, predicted a significant, but small, portion of variance in depression. However, both dimensions of psychological abuse (i.e., dominance/isolation, emotional/verbal), taken separately predicted approximately 20% of the variance in depression. Further, while Campbell and colleagues' research found that nonphysical abuse made no significant contribution to the multivariate prediction of depression, the present study found the opposite where it was only psychological—and not physical—abuse that predicted depression. While Campbell and associates' research included measures of childhood abuse and tangible resources, the present study did not. Further, the present study was specific to a justice system context, whereas Campbell and colleagues used a sample recruited from the community through newspaper and bulletin board advertisements. Nevertheless, it is as yet unclear how these differences may explain the varied results.

In sum, this study supports the conclusion that measures of both psychological and physical abuse should be included routinely in studies of battered women's response to violence and domestic violence generally. Physical abuse variables played a more significant role in battered women's use of the legal system and in leaving the abusive relationship but psychological abuse variables play a more important role in predicting battered women's traumatic response to violence.

REFERENCES

Ascione, F. R. (1998). Battered women's reports of their partner's and their children's cruelty to animals. *Journal of Emotional Abuse, 1*(1), 119-133.

Belle, D. (1982). Social ties and social support. In D. Belle (Ed.), *Lives in stress: Women in depression* (pp. 133-144). Beverly Hills, CA: Sage.

Brown, J. (1997). Working toward freedom from violence: The process of change in battered women. *Violence Against Women, 3*(1), 5-26.

Campbell, J. C., Kub, J., Belknap, R. A., & Templin, T. N. (1997). Predictors of depression in battered women. *Violence Against Women, 3*(3), 271-293.

Campbell, J. C., & Lewandowski, L. A. (1997). Mental and physical health effects of intimate partner violence on women and children. *Psychiatric Clinics of North America, 20*(2), 353-374.

Carbone, P. M. (1996). *Psychological abuse and the battered woman.* Nova Southeastern University, Ft. Lauderdale.

Cardena, E. (1996). Psychometric review of the Stanford Acute Stress Reaction Questionnaire (SASRQ). In B. H. Stamm (Ed.), *Measurement of stress, trauma, and adaptation.* Lutherville, MD: Sidran Press.

Cascardi, M., & O'Leary, K. D. (1992). Depressive symptomatology, self-esteem, and self-blame in battered women. *Journal of Family Violence, 7*(4), 249-259.

Dutton, M. A. (1993). Understanding women's responses to domestic violence: A redefinition of battered woman syndrome. *Hofstra Law Review, 21*(4), 1191-1242.

Dutton, M. A. (1996). Battered women's strategic response to violence: The role of context. In J. L. E. Z. C. Eisikovits (Ed.), *Future interventions with battered women and their families* (pp. 105-124). Thousand Oaks, CA: Sage Publications.

Fischer, K., Campbell, R., & Rappaport, J. (in press). The effect of resource availability on battered women's decision to follow through with court orders of protection.

Foa, E. B., Riggs, D. S., Dancu, C., & Rothbaum, B. O. (1993). Reliability and validity of a brief instrument for assessing PTSD. *Journal of Traumatic Stress, 6,* 459-473.

194   *Interrelationships and Outcomes*

Follingstad, D. R., Brenan, A. F., Hause, E. S., Polek, D. S., & Rutledge, L. L. (1991). Factors moderating physical and psychological symptoms of battered women. *Journal of Family Violence, 6*(1), 81-95.

Follingstad, D. R., Rutledge, L. L., Berg, B. J., Hause, E. S., & Polek, D. S. (1990). The role of emotional abuse in physically abusive relationships. *Journal of Family Violence, 5*(2), 107-120.

Ganley, A. (1989). Integrating feminist and social learning analyses of aggression: Creating multiple models for intervention with men who battered. In P. Caesar & L. Hamberger (Eds.), *Treating men who batter* (pp. 196-235). New York: Springer Publishing.

Gondolf, E. W., & Fisher, E. R. (1988). *Battered women as survivors: An alternative to treating learned helplessness.* Lexington, MA: Lexington Books.

Gondolf, E. W., McWilliams, J., Hart, B., & Stuehling, J. (1994). Court responses for petitions for civil protection orders. *Journal of Interpersonal Violence, 9*(4), 503-517.

Goodman, L., Bennett, L., & Dutton, M. A. (in press). Factors related to domestic violence victims' cooperation with criminal prosecution of their abuser:The role of social support. *Violence and Victims.*

Goodman, L. A. (1991). The prevalence of abuse among homeless and housed poor mothers: A comparison study. *American Journal of Orthopsychiatry, 61*(4), 489-500.

Gortner, E., Jacobson, N. S., Berns, S. B., & Gottman, J. M. (1997). When women leave violent relationships: Dispelling clinical myths. *Psychotherapy, 34*(4), 343-352.

Harrell, A., Smith, B., & Newmark, L. (1993). *Court processing and the effects of restraining orders for domestic violence victims.* Washington, DC: The Urban Institute.

Houskamp, B. M., & Foy, D. M. (1991). The assessment of posttraumatic stress disorder in battered women. *Journal of Interpersonal Violence, 6*(3), 367-375.

Hudson, W. W., & McIntosh, S. R. (1981). The assessment of spouse abuse: Two quantifiable dimensions. *Journal of Marriage and the Family, 43,* 873-885.

Hutchinson, I. W., & Ahirschel, J. D. (1998). Abused women: Help-seeking strategies and police utilization. *Violence Against Women, 4*(4), 436-456.

Jacobson, N. S., Gottman, J. M., Gortner, E., Berns, S., & Shortt, J. W. (1996). Psychological factors in the longitudinal course of battering: When do the couples split up? When does the abuse decrease? *Violence and Victims, 11*(4), 371-392.

Kantor, G. K., & Straus, M. A. (1990). Response of victims and the police to assaults on wives. In M. A. Straus & R. J. Gelles (Eds.), *Physical violence in American families* (pp. 473-487). New Brunswick.

Kaslow, N. J., Thompson, M. P., Meadows, L. A., Jacobs, D., Chance, S., Gibb, B., Bornsein, H., Hollins, L., Rashid, A., & Phillips, K. (1998). Factors that mediate and moderate the link between partner abuse and suicidal behavior in African American women. *Journal of Consulting and Clinical Psychology, 66*(3), 533-540.

Keilitz, S. L., Hannaford, P. L., & Efkeman, H. S. (1997). *Civil protection orders: The benefits and limitations for victims of domestic violence.* Williamsburg, VA: National Center for State Courts.

Kemp, A., Green, B. L., Horowitz, C., & Rawlins, E. I. (1995). Incidence and correlates of PTSD in battered women: Shelter and community samples. *Journal of Interpersonal Violence, 10*(1), 43-55.

Marshall, L. L. (1996). Psychological abuse of women: Six distinct clusters. *Journal of Family Violence, 11*(4), 379-409.

Radloff, L. S. (1977). The CES-D scale: A self-report depression scale for research in the general population. *Applied Psychological Measurement, 1*(3), 385-401.

Rebovich, D. J. (1996). Prosecution response to domestic violence: Results of a survey of large jurisdictions. In E. S. Buzawa & C. G. Buzawa (Eds.), *Do arrests and restraining orders work* (pp. 176-191). Thousand Oaks, CA: Sage.

Rusbult, C. E., & Martz, J. M. (1995). Remaining in an abusive relationship: An investment model analysis of nonvoluntary dependence. *Personality & Social Psychology Bulletin, 21*(6), 558-571.

Spiegel, D., Koopman, C., Classen, C., & Cardena, E. *The development of a state measure of dissociative reactions to trauma.* (Final report to the NIMH). Stanford University.

Stark, E. (1995). Re-presenting woman battering: From battered woman syndrome to coercive control. *Albany Law Review, 58,* 973-1026.

Straus, M. A., Hamby, S. L., Boney-McCoy, S., & Sugarman, D. B. (1995). *The Revised Conflicts Tactics Scales* (CTS-2). Durham, NH: Family Research Laboratory.

Strube, M. (1988). The decision to leave an abusive relationship: Empirical evidence and theoretical issues. *Psychological Bulletin, 104,* 236-250.

Tolman, R. (1989). The development of a measure of psychological maltreatment of women by their male partners. *Violence and Victims, 4*(3), 173-189.

Tolman, R. (1999). The validation of the Psychological Maltreatment of Women Inventory. *Violence and Victims, 14,* 25-37.

Tuel, B. D., & Russell, R. K. (1998). Self-esteem and depression in battered women. *Violence Against Women, 4*(3), 34-362.

van der Kolk, B., McFarlane, A. C., & Weisaeth, L. (1996). *Traumatic stress.* New York: The Guilford Press.

Weaver, T. L., & Clum, G. A. (1995). Psychological distress associated with interpersonal violence: A metal-analyses. *Clinical Psychology Review, 15*(2), 115-140.

Wilson, J. P., & Raphael, B. (1993). *International handbook of traumatic stress syndromes.* New York: Plenum Press.

Chapter 11

The Impact of Different Forms of Psychological Abuse on Battered Women

Leslie A. Sackett and Daniel G. Saunders

P ractitioners and researchers are paying increasing attention to the psychological abuse of women (Follingstad, Rutledge, Berg, Hause, & Polek, 1990; Loring, 1994; Tolman, 1989). A major reason for this focus is the realization that psychological abuse may be just as detrimental, or more detrimental, than physical abuse. In one study, 72% of the battered women reported that emotional abuse had a more severe impact than physical abuse (Follingstad et al., 1990). In another study, psychological abuse was more strongly associated with psychosocial problems than threats or physical abuse (Tolman & Bhosley, 1991). The focus of most previous work is on women who are both physically and psychologically abused. Almost all women who are physically abused also report verbal abuse (83%; Walker, 1984) or psychological abuse (99%; Follingstad et al., 1990). Another reason to focus on psychological abuse is the evidence that verbal aggression early in the relationship is a frequent precursor of physical aggression later (Murphy & O'Leary, 1989). Thus, identifying particular forms of psychological abuse may help prevent physical abuse later in the relationship.

Psychological abuse can also help to maintain abusive relationships. If severe enough, it may lead to self-doubt, confusion, and depression. Battered women may subsequently have a difficult time seeing their options and marshaling the resources needed to leave the relationship. At first, a battered woman may respond to criticism and put-downs by trying to change herself, convince her partner they need couple's counseling, or attribute his abuse to his drinking. Over time, many women realize that nothing they do seems to make a difference. Women may be especially affected by emotional abuse coming from a significant other because of the importance of mutuality to their psychological development (Miller, 1991). Qualitative research on battered women finds that battered women may experience a loss of identity directly related to coerced isolation, emotional abuse and "acts of diminishment" (Larkin & Popaleni, 1994; Mills, 1985; Smith, Tessaro, & Earp, 1995).

Along with the increased attention currently given to psychological abuse have come attempts to classify the various forms that it takes. Direct practice work with battered women and men who batter helped to create lists of a broad range of abusive behaviors (e.g., NiCarthy, 1982; Pence & Paymar, 1993; Sonkin, Martin, & Walker, 1985). Some practitioners drew parallels between battered women and prisoners of war, and thus the lists included techniques that are commonly used in brainwashing: degradation and threats with occasional indulgences, isolation, and invalidation of perceptions (Walker, 1984). Survey research that built on these observations and classifications has pointed to a number of different types. Tolman (1989) factor-analyzed 58 forms of psychological maltreatment and found two major dimensions: dominance-isolation and emotional-verbal. Aguilar and Nightingale (1994) divided abuse into "controlling/emotional" and "sexual/emotional," based on their cluster analysis. Using semistructured interviews, Follingstad and her colleagues (1990) created a list of five types: threats of abuse, ridicule; jealousy; threats to change marriage; restriction; and damage to property. Marshall (1996) uncovered six patterns of psychological abuse through a cluster analysis of a large sample. The patterns were as follows: (1) severe violence but without denigration or control of finances; (2) moderate violence and sexual abuse; (3) low on abuse but enforced isolation; (4) low levels of violence with overt criticism and several types of control; (5) several types of overtly dominating and controlling abuse and lower levels of sexual aggression; and (6) similar to cluster 5 but with different patterns of help-seeking.

Few attempts have been made to discover the forms of psychological abuse that have the most severe impacts. The women in Follingstad and colleagues' (1990) study reported that ridicule was the worst form. In the Aguilar and Nightingale study (1994), women who experienced "controlling/emotional" abuse had lower self-esteem scores. Dutton and Painter (1993) found that dominance/isolation was more strongly related to trauma and low self-esteem than emotional-verbal abuse 6 months after the abuse occurred.

The purpose of this study was to extend previous research on the different types of psychological abuse experienced by battered women and to examine whether some types of psychological abuse are rated as more severe than others. We predicted that, similar to the study by Follingstad and her associates (Follingstad et al., 1990), ridiculing of traits would be rated as more severe because it attacks a person's sense of self more directly than other types of abuse. For example, if a woman's behavior is criticized she may believe that she needs to change specific behaviors. Her hope for the relationship may continue and she is less likely to become depressed (Frieze, 1978). Ridiculing of her traits, however—an attack on her character—is more likely to shatter her sense of hope, security in the relationship, and even her sense of self. Depression, low self-esteem and further alienation and isolation from herself and others is likely to result. In our test of this hypothesis, we went beyond simple severity ratings to assess the impact of psychological abuse on distinct outcomes: depression, self-esteem, and fear.

We used more extensive measures of abuse and its impact than most other studies and therefore hoped to explore more fully questions about the impact of various forms of psychological abuse on battered women. Furthermore, we wanted to know if psychological abuse acts independently of physical abuse on depression, self-esteem, and fear, and if so, to what extent. Given the large overlap between physical and psychological abuse, it seems important to partial the effects of physical abuse from that of psychological abuse.

We also wanted to explore whether sheltered and nonsheltered women differ on levels of psychological abuse. Sheltered women generally suffer more severe physical abuse (e.g., Wilson, Vercella, Brems, Benning, & Renfro, 1992) and the pattern may be the same for psychological abuse. However, the two forms of abuse do not always correlate (e.g., Sabourin, 1991).

METHOD

Respondents

Respondents had sought help from a domestic violence agency in a midsized midwestern city. All of the women had been physically abused at least once. Thirty women were shelter residents and 30 were in nonresidential individual or group counseling for domestic violence. Average age was 34.7 years. ($SD = 9.1$). The majority of the women were White (62%); 30% were African American and 5% were Native American. One woman was Hispanic and one was Asian. Most of the women (63%) had some college and 25% were college graduates. Forty percent were employed full-time and 25% part-time. Most of the women (62%) had children ($M = 1.2$; $SD = 1.2$). Seventy percent of the women were currently living with their partners. The majority of partners were spouses (56%).

Procedure

Data collection took place over a 9 month period. Routine intake forms required by the state social service department provided some information for the study, such as demographics and abuse history. Other information was collected through an interview designed for the study. The women in the shelter were recruited by a staff member who gave the women information about the study a day or 2 after they entered the shelter. Following informed consent procedures, an interviewer was assigned to the woman. During the period that the 30 sheltered women were interviewed, 45 other women were sheltered. Many of these women were not interviewed because they left the shelter before an interview could be arranged.

The women who were not sheltered were recruited by their individual ($n = 18$) or group counselor ($n = 12$). When counselors wanted to refer a woman, information about the study was given to her and she completed informed consent procedures. The interviewers, trained by the first author, were staff members ($n = 2$) or volunteers ($n = 5$) of the domestic violence agency or undergraduates majoring in psychology ($n = 3$). The first author interviewed 21 of the women. The interviews lasted approximately 11/2 hours, but ranged from 1.25 hours to 3.5 hours. Fifteen of these women had never left their partners, 3 had stayed at a shelter at some time, and the remaining 12 stayed temporarily or permanently with friends, relatives, or on their own. Many of the women were referred to a special group for partners of men who were in treatment. Other women were referred by agencies, friends or themselves.

Measures

Depression. The Beck Depression Inventory (BDI)(Beck, 1967) was used to measure depression. The BDI contains 21 items that cover mood, guilt, loss of interest, and physical signs. It has good concurrent and construct validity (Beck, 1967). The internal reliability coefficient (alpha) in this study was .90.

Self-esteem. This construct was measured with a version of the Coopersmith Self-esteem Inventory (Coopersmith, 1967) designed for a general population. The scale contains 25 items with a response format of "like me" or "unlike me." The internal reliability coefficient (alpha) in this study was .90. It is demonstrated to have good convergent and discriminant validity (Johnson, Redfield, Miller, & Simpson, 1983).

Fear. A 6-item scale of battered women's fear was constructed for this study. Originally, 14 items were constructed and administered. The scale was reduced to 6-items through item analysis and by choosing items which clearly described emotional impact. The 6-item version had an internal reliability coefficient (alpha) of .86 which was higher than the 14-item version (see Appendix). The response format was: "never, less than once a month, once a month, 2–3 times a month, once a week, 2–3 times a week, and daily."

Profile of Psychological Abuse. This measure was developed for the study based on earlier work (Sackett, 1992). It initially contained 42 items drawn from clinical work, descriptions of the tactics of men who batter (Pence & Paymar, 1993), and the experiences of battered women as categorized by NiCarthy (1982). The items covered a wide variety of psychological abuse: humiliation, threats, invalidation of experiences, isolation, trivial demands, occasional indulgences, and emotional distance. The response format was the same as for the fear scale: "never, less than once a month, once a month, 2–3 times a month, once a week, 2–3 times a week, and daily." Seven items were removed because of ambiguous wording. The remaining 35 items were entered into a principal component factor analysis with varimax rotation. A scree test revealed that a 5-factor solution was optimal. All 5-factors were interpretable. One factor of 6 items was not retained because it did not reflect behaviors that were clearly abusive. As evidence for this, it did not correlate significantly with the womens' depression and low self-esteem.

Eight other items were deleted in order to improve the reliability of the subscales. The factor analysis was repeated with the 21-item version and the factor structure was consistent with the original analysis with 35 items with the exception of one item. The final 21 items are shown in the Appendix, along with the item-factor loadings and the internal alpha coefficients of the subscales. The factors were labeled as follows: Jealous Control (alpha = .85); Ignore (alpha = .80); Ridicule Traits (alpha = .79); and Criticize Behavior (alpha = .75).

Severity of Psychological Abuse. A single question asked about the severity level of abuse: "Overall, how would you rate the severity of the psychological abuse?" (not severe at all, mildly severe, very severe, extremely severe).

Demographics. Age, educational level (five levels), and income (nine levels) were taken from intake forms.

Violence. The intake form contained four questions on violence, with the first two requiring yes or no responses—Did the assailant use any of the following: a gun? a knife, or other cutting instrument? hands/fist/feet? sexual assault? threats to kill?; Did the client ever receive any of the following injuries from the assailant: cuts/burns/ bruises? choking? internal injuries? strains/sprains/broken bones? head injuries? How often does any of the violence occur: never, once a year or less, approximately 3–4 times a year, approximately once a month, approximately once a week, almost daily; Length of time the client has been exposed to abuse by the assailant: no previous abuse, less than 1 year, 1 to 3 years, 3 to 5 years, more than 5 years.

Based on a factor analysis (principal component with varimax rotation) of the violence and injury items, the items "fist/feet/hands" and "cuts/burns/bruises" were labeled as "moderate violence" and all the rest as "severe violence." A variable called "Amount of Violence" was constructed by giving a double weight to the severe items, adding them to the less severe items and multiplying the total by the frequency of violence. An advantage of multiplying severity by frequency is that a more normal distribution is approached than when either variable is used alone. The item on the duration of violence in the relationship was kept intact.

Relationship Happiness. This construct was measured with items from a measure of relationship satisfaction developed by Veroff (1988). A factor analysis revealed one factor out of five that could clearly be labeled "relationship satisfaction." The highest loading items were: (1) "Would you say your relationship is: not too happy, just about average, a little happier than average, very happy?"; (2) "When you think about your relationship—what each of you puts into it, and gets out of it—how happy do you feel?"; (3) "When you think about your relationship—what each of you puts into it, and gets out of it—how angry do you feel?"; (4) "How stable do you feel your relationship is?"; and (5) "All in all, how satisfied are you with your relationship?" The response format was on a four point scale from "never" to "often." Factor scores were used in the analysis in order to use weighted items. The internal alpha coefficient of reliability was .78.

Analysis

We used a t-test to compare the sheltered and nonsheltered women on abuse and demographic variables. Hierarchical multiple regression analysis was used to test the relative impact of psychological and physical abuse on depression, self-esteem, and fear.

RESULTS

Compared with the women who had not been in the shelter, the sheltered women had less education and income and experienced more severe physical abuse (see Table 1). They also had higher scores on two of the psychological abuse scales: Ridicule Traits and Jealous Control (Table 1). Despite more physical and psychological abuse among the sheltered women, they did not have higher scores on depression and fear or lower scores on self-esteem. The average score for both groups of women on the Beck Depression Inventory was 18.1 ($SD = 12.5$), which is in the moderate range. There was considerable variation on this measure: 30% scored as nondepressed (0–9), 27% as mildly depressed (10–18), 27% as moderately depressed (19–29), and 17% as severely depressed (30 or over) (norms from Beck, Steer, & Garbin, 1988).

Table 2 shows the relationship among the independent and dependent variables for both groups of women combined. As predicted, psychological abuse severity was much more strongly related to ridiculing of traits than criticism of behavior. Psychological abuse severity also showed a significant but weak correlation with "jealous control." In addition, severity correlated positively with the amount of violence and fear and negatively with relationship satisfaction.

In the prediction of depression, the strongest bivariate correlation was with the amount of violence, followed by the global severity rating of psychological abuse. Ignoring and ridiculing of traits were also significantly related to depression. Unexpectedly, the duration of violence was negatively related to depression. The amount of violence also had the highest correlations with low self-esteem, followed

**Table 1. Mean Comparisons of Sheltered and Nonsheltered
Battered Women on Abuse and Demographic Variables
(Standard Deviation in Parentheses)**

	Sheltered $n = 30$	Nonsheltered $n = 30$	t
Psychological Abuse			
Ridicule Her Traits	24.6	20.4	2.08*
	(7.1)	(8.1)	
Jealous Control	40.7	31.7	2.95*
	(11.1)	(12.4)	
Criticize Behavior	9.8	9.8	.00
	(6.1)	(5.7)	
Ignore	22.5	23.3	-.34
	(9.2)	(8.5)	
Overall Frequency	5.5	5.6	-.49
	(0.8)	(0.8)	
Overall Severity	3.1	3.1	.00
	(0.8)	(0.8)	
Physical Abuse			
Severe Violence	4.9	3.2	2.79**
Duration	4.1	4.1	.12
Demographics			
Age	34.4	34.9	-.21
Education	3.2	4.1	-3.19**
Household Income	5.0	7.3	-3.73***

*$p < .05$; **$p < .01$; ***$p < .001$.

by ignoring. Ridiculing of traits was also significantly related to lower self-esteem. Relationships with the fear of abuse were the strongest. Ridiculing of traits was the most strongly related to fear. Jealous/control, criticizing behavior, ignoring, and the amount of violence all had moderately high correlations with fearfulness.

Although Jealous/Control had relatively low correlations with depression and self-esteem, it had the highest correlation with physical abuse, compared with the other forms of psychological abuse (ave. $r = .32$).

The three dependent variables, depression, self-esteem, and fear, were correlated with each other in expected directions. Depression and low self-esteem were the most highly correlated.

The correlation matrices (six independent and three dependent variables) were compared between the two samples. Fifteen of the 18 correlations were similar. Sheltered women had much higher correlations between "ignore" and depression and self-esteem; and violence duration and depression.

Table 3 shows the results of the hierarchical multiple regression in the prediction of depression, self-esteem, and fear. Psychological abuse and violence variables were entered in separate blocks. Psychological abuse was entered first, followed by

Table 2. Correlations Among the Dependent and Independent Variables

	1	2	3	4	5	6	7	8	9	10	11
1. Fear	—	-.25*	.29**	.56***	.47***	.66***	.52*	.31**	.01	.42***	-.34**
2. Self-Esteem			-.65***	-.17	-.31**	-.22*	-.17	-.08	.05	-.34**	.05
3. Depression				.18	.22*	.23*	.20	.31**	-.23*	.34**	-.40***
4. Jealous/Control					.33**	.53***	.43***	.23*	-.15	.49***	-.24*
5. Ignore						.47***	.55***	.17	-.03	.26*	-.16
6. Ridicule traits							.54***	.55***	.13	.36**	-.42***
7. Criticize behavior								.17	.35**	-.12	
8. Global severity of psychological abuse									-.04	.36**	-.61***
9. Duration of violence										.07	.16
10. Amount of violence											-.22*
11. Relationship satisfaction											—

$*p < .05; **p < .01; ***p < .001.$

violence. The procedure was then reversed with violence entered first. In this way, the unique variance of psychological versus physical abuse could be determined.

Jealous/Control was not entered into the first two equations because it had the lowest correlation of the psychological abuse variables with depression and self-esteem and the sample was too small for using all of the variables. The psychological abuse variables accounted for 13% of the variance in depression. When the physical abuse variables were entered, the variance accounted for rose significantly by 10%. When the order was reversed, the violence variables accounted for 18% of the variance, showing a (not quite significant) 5% increase with the addition of the psychological abuse variables. Thus, psychological abuse and physical abuse made unique contributions in explaining depression, with a somewhat stronger contribution by physical abuse.

In the prediction of self-esteem, the variance accounted for when the psychological abuse variables were entered was 10%; with the addition of the violence variables, it rose significantly by 9%. When the violence variables were entered first, they accounted for 12% of the variance in predicting self-esteem; the addition of psychological abuse significantly increased the variance explained by 7%. Once again, psychological and physical abuse made independent contributions to the outcome variable.

In the prediction of fear, the global severity rating of psychological abuse was dropped from the equation. Although it was significantly related to fear ($r = .31$), the four types of psychological abuse were much more strongly related to it (ave. $r = .55$). The psychological abuse variables accounted for 53% of the variance. The

Table 3. Hierarchical Multiple Regression

	Dependent Variable		
Independent Variable	Depression	Self-Esteem	Fear
Step 1: Psychological Abuse			
$R =$	.37	.32	.73
$R^2 =$	.13	.10	.53
Step 2: Violence			
$R =$	.48	.43	.73
$R^2 =$	.23	.19	.54
R square increase =	.10	.09	.01
F for increase =	7.40**	6.33**	1.24
Step 1: Violence			
$R =$	.43	.34	.42
$R^2 =$	.18	.12	.18
Step 2: Psychological Abuse			
$R =$	.48	.43	.73
$R^2 =$	.23	.19	.54
R square increase =	.05	.07	.36
F for increase =	3.70	4.93**	44.6***

$*p < .05; **p < .01; ***p < .001.$

entry of the physical abuse variables added only 1% to the variance. When the physical abuse variables were entered first, they accounted for 18% of the variance. The addition of the psychological abuse variables raised the percent variance by 36%, a very significant increase. Thus, psychological abuse was a much stronger predictor of fear than physical abuse.

DISCUSSION

The factor analysis of the Profile of Psychological Abuse revealed four major forms of abuse: Criticize Behavior, Ignore, Ridicule Traits, and Jealous/Control (Appendix). The Jealous/Control factor appears similar to the Dominance-Isolation factor of Tolman's (1989) Psychological Maltreatment of Women Inventory (PMWI), which also included items on jealousy and restriction of behavior. It also has items similar to the Controlling/Emotional Abuse items from the Aguilar and Nightingale study (1994). The Ignore factor has items similar to some of those on the Emotional-Verbal subscale of the PMWI (e.g., "sulked, refused to talk," "withheld affection"). The Criticize Behavior factor seemed closer to items on the Dominance-Isolation factor of the PMWI, whereas the Ridicule Traits factor seemed closer to items on the Emotional-Verbal factor of the PMWI. However, these similarities were not clear-cut.

An important feature of the Profile of Psychological Abuse is its ability to distinguish between criticism of behaviors and ridiculing of traits. It also has the advantage of using specific time referents (e.g., "once a month,," "once a week," "2-3 times a week," etc.). The differing patterns of psychological abuse found in this and other studies probably reflect the behavior of different types of men who batter. Some men seem to restrict their partners' behavior out of jealousy, while others tend to blame their partners for the violence, treat them as inferiors, and use threats (Holtzworth-Munroe & Stuart, 1994). Battered women's experiences can also be clustered into different groups depending on the types of violence they experienced and their causal attributions for the violence (Follingstad, Laughlin, Polek, Rutledge, & Hause, 1991; Snyder & Fruchtman, 1981).

Battered women residing in a shelter reported more severe physical abuse. This finding is consistent with other studies (Saunders, 1994; Wilson et al., 1992), as are the findings that the sheltered women had less education and income. These women also experienced more ridicule of their personal characteristics and jealous control by their partners. Surprisingly, their depression, self-esteem, and fear did not differ from nonsheltered battered women. The shelter may have provided enough support in a short period of time for previous depression and fear to lift. Self-esteem is less likely to change in such a short period of time. However, one study found that the length of stay in a shelter was related to higher self-esteem and lower depression (Orava, McLeod, & Sharpe, 1996).

Another possibility is that the more severe abuse experienced by these women produced traumatic symptoms , such as "numbing" and dissociative responses, that kept other emotional responses from surfacing. The fight for survival and the recency of abuse might not have allowed them to feel depressed or fearful, at least for the time immediately after the abuse. Other research shows that sheltered women have more frequent symptoms of posttraumatic stress than other help-seeking battered women (Gleason, 1993; Saunders, 1994).

The average level of depression on the BDI for both samples was somewhat below that of another sample of battered women. In that sample 33% of the women were in the severe range (score over 30)(Orava, McLeod, & Sharpe, 1996).

As predicted, ridiculing of traits was related most strongly to the severity rating of psychological abuse. The other forms of psychological abuse, especially criticizing behavior and ignoring, are somewhat less likely to be taken personally. Jealous-controlling behavior, although most strongly related to the amount of physical abuse, might be viewed as a less severe form of psychological abuse for the same reason: it is not a direct attack on the self. Similarly, there was no relation between jealous/control and depression. Again, the women might be able to make external attributions, i.e., to readily see through the tactics and jealousy of their partners without blaming themselves. These findings are consistent with the distinction made between behavioral self-blame and characterological self-blame that Janoff-Bulman (1982) applied to rape survivors. Behavioral blame is a less severe form of blame and provides the victim with a sense of control that "there is something about myself that I can change to prevent an attack." These forms of attributions are less likely to have an impact on depression and self-esteem (Frieze, 1978). Jealous/control may also have been interpreted positively by many of these women, just has it does for many college women (Henton, Cate, Koval, Lloyd, & Christopher, 1983). At least early in the relationship, jealousy may be viewed as a sign of romantic love.

This study revealed that psychological and physical abuse had fairly independent effects on depression and self-esteem. However, psychological abuse had a much stronger impact than physical abuse on fear. Ridiculing traits, criticizing behavior, and jealous/control had the strongest relationship to fear. The intimidating behavior of the most controlling type of batterer may be partly responsible for the greater fear. The amount of physical abuse, but not its duration, was also significantly related to fear.

Depression was related to criticism, ignoring, ridicule, and violence as expected. The negative relation between depression and the duration of violence is more difficult to explain. It is possible that women experiencing the most severe violence had shorter relationships; those experiencing less severe violence might have been able to find ways to keep their hope alive and keep their depression lower. Alternately, as with the speculation we made about the severe trauma to sheltered women, the survival needs of those enduring long-term abuse may cause numbing and a suppression of feelings.

The amount of violence and ignoring were most strongly related to low self-esteem. The act of violence itself gives the message that the victim is unworthy and unlovable. In one study of the men's accounts, many of the men admitted that they were trying to convince their wives that they were worthless through a combination of verbal and physical abuse (Hyden, 1995). The finding on the use of ignoring shows that it needs to be taken seriously as a form of abuse, with the potential for long-term consequences. Being ignored may give one of the most negative messages possible about self-worth.

For practitioners, these results confirm the negative impact that psychological abuse has on battered women's emotional life and sense of self. Practitioners can help women to see why "character assassinations" are more devastating than specific criticisms, but also why specific criticisms might build unrealistic hopes. Ignoring needs to be discussed as an extreme form of abuse because it conveys the message: "you don't exist." Group work is particularly well suited to help battered women overcome psychological abuse because they can learn that their experiences are similar to those of other women, their experiences and emotions can be validated by others, and mutual support can occur. There is some evidence that such group work not only increases self-esteem and a sense of inner control but also may help to reduce psychological abuse (Tutty, Bidgood, & Rothery, 1993).

The conclusions of this study need to be viewed cautiously due to a number of limitations. The sample was relatively small and all of the women were seeking help. Not all of the women who were asked to participate were willing or able to do so. Nonparticipants tended to be those who left the shelter more quickly and were probably less traumatized. The results may also differ with nonhelp-seeking samples. The measure of physical aggression was derived from an intake form and had unknown reliability and validity. If it was less reliable than the psychological abuse variables, the relationship between physical abuse and the outcome variables would be attenuated. The measures of psychological abuse and fear were developed for this study. Although showing adequate scale reliability, tests of validity outside of the hypotheses of this study were not available. All of these limitations point the way for future research.

Despite these limitations, this study shows the utility of a new measure of psychological abuse. The findings suggest that the psychic injuries to battered women are typically caused as much by psychological abuse as physical abuse. Some forms of psychological abuse appear more damaging than others. With the replication of these results, counseling methods can be refined and tested for countering what are probably the most lingering effects of woman abuse—those which affect the survivor's very sense of self.

REFERENCES

Aguilar, R. J., & Nightingale, N. N. (1994). The impact of specific battering experiences on the self-esteem of abused women. *Journal of Family Violence, 9,* 35-46.

Beck, A. T. (1967). *Depression: Clinical, experimental and theoretical aspects.* New York: Harper & Row.

Beck, A. T., Steer, R. A., & Garbin, M. G. (1988). Psychometric properties of the Beck Depression Inventory. *Clinical Psychology Review, 8,* 77-100.

Coopersmith, S. (1967). *Self-esteem inventories.* Palo Alto, CA: Consulting Psychology Press.

Dutton, D. G., & Painter, S. (1993). Emotional attachment in abusive relationships. *Violence and Victims, 8,* 105-120.

Follingstad, D. R., Laughlin, J. E., Polek, D. S., Rutledge, L. L., & Hause, E. S. (1991). Identification of patterns of wife abuse. *Journal of Interpersonal Violence, 6,* 187-204.

Follingstad, D. R., Rutledge, L., Polek, D., & McNeill-Hawkins, K. (1988). Factors associated with patterns of dating violence toward college women. *Journal of Family Violence, 3,* 169-182.

Follingstad, D. R., Rutledge, L. L, Berg, B. J., Hause, E. S., & Polek, D. S. (1990). The role of emotional abuse in physically abusive relationships. *Journal of Family Violence, 5,* 107-120.

Frieze, I. H. (1978). *New approaches to social problems.* San Francisco: Jossey-Bass.

Gleason, W. J. (1993). Mental Disorders in battered women: An empirical study. *Violence & Victims, 8,* 53-68.

Henton, J., Cate, R., Koval, J., Lloyd, S., & Christopher, S. (1983). Romance and violence in dating relationships. *Journal of Family Issues, 4,* 467-482.

Holtzworth-Munroe, A., & Stuart, G. L. (1994). Typologies of male batterers: Three subtypes and the differences among them. *Psychological Bulletin, 116,* 476-497.

Hyden, M. (1995). Verbal aggression as prehistory of woman battering. *Journal of Family Violence, 10,* 55-73.

Janoff-Bulman, R. (1982). Esteem and control bases of blame: "Adaptive" strategies for victim versus observers. *Journal of Personality, 30,* 180-192.

Johnson, B. W., Redfield, D. L., Miller, R., & Simpson, R. E. (1983). The Coopersmith Self-Esteem Inventory: A construct validity study. *Educational and Psychological Measurement,* 907-913.

Larkin, J., & Popaleni, K. (1994). Heterosexual courtship violence and sexual harassment: The private and public control of young women. *Feminism & Psychology, 4,* 213-227.

Loring, M. T (1994) *Emotional abuse.* New York: Lexington Books.

Marshall, L. (1996). Psychological abuse of women: Six distinct clusters. *Journal of Family Violence, 11,* 379-410.

Miller, J. B. (1991). The development of women's sense of self. In J. V. Jordan et al., (Eds.), *Women's growth through connection.* New York: Guilford.

Mills, T. (1985). The assault on the self: Stages in coping with battering husbands. *Qualitative Sociology, 8,* 103-123.

Murphy, C., & O'Leary, K. D. (1989). Psychological aggression predicts physical aggression in early marriage. *Journal of Consulting and Clinical Psychology, 57,* 579-582.

NiCarthy, G. (1982). *Getting free: A handbook for women in abusive relationships.* Seattle: Seal Press.

Orava, T. A, McLeod, P. J., & Sharpe, D. (1996). Perceptions of control, depressive symptomatology, and self-esteem of women in transition from abusive relationships. *Journal of Family Violence, 11,* 167-186.

Pence, E., & Paymar, M. (1993). *Education groups for men who batter.* New York: Springer Publishing.

Sabourin, T. C. (1991). Perceptions of verbal aggression in interpersonal violence. In D. D. Knudsen & J. L. Miller (Eds.), *Abused and battered.* New York: Aldine de Gruyter.

Sackett, L. A. (1992). Assessing psychological abuse among battered women. Unpublished dissertation, University of Michigan, School of Social Work and Department of Psychology, Ann Arbor, MI.

Saunders, D. G. (1994). Posttraumatic stress symptom profiles of battered women: A comparison of survivors in two settings. *Violence and Victims, 9,* 125-138.

Sonkin, D. J., Martin, D., & Walker, L. E. A. (1985). *The male batterer: A treatment approach.* New York: Springer Publishing.

Smith, P. H., Tessaro, I., & Earp, J. A. L. (1995). Women's experiences with battering: A conceptualization from qualitative research. *Women's Health Issues, 5,* 173-182.

Snyder, D. K., & Fruchtman, L. A. (1981). Differential patterns of wife abuse: A data-based typology. *Journal of Consulting and Clinical Psychology, 49,* 878-885.

Tolman, R. M. (1989). The development of a measure of psychological maltreatment of women by their male partners. *Violence and Victims, 4,* 159-178.

Tolman, R. M., & Bhosley, G. (1991). The outcome of participation in a shelter-sponsored program for men who batter. In D. Knudsen & J. Miller (Eds.), *Abused and Battered: Social and Legal Responses.* New York: Aldine de Gruyter.

Tutty, L. M., Bidgood, B. A., & Rothery, M. A. (1993). Support groups for battered women: Research on their efficacy. *Journal of Family Violence, 8,* 325-344.

Veroff, J. (1988). First years of marriage: Wave III: Spouse questionnaire. Survey Research Center, Institute for Social Research. University of Michigan, Ann Arbor, MI.

Walker, L. E. (1984). *The battered woman syndrome.* New York: Springer Publishing.

Wilson, K, Vercella, R., Brems, C., Benning, D., & Renfro, N. (1992). Levels of learned helplessness in abused women. *Women & Therapy, 13,* 53-67.

APPENDIX
Profile of Psychological Abuse

As much as possible, I would like you to disregard the physical abuse that has occurred in your current relationship. The question I am asking should be answered according to the psychological or emotional abuse that has occurred in your relationship. I know some of these questions may be hard to answer, but please try to be as accurate as possible.
Response format under each item:

1	2	3	4	5	6	7
never	less than once	once a month	2–3 times a month	once a week	2–3 times a week	daily

Jealous Control
Internal Alpha Reliability = .85

Factor
Loading
.74 Become angry or upset if you want to be with someone else and not with him?
.70 Intercept your mail, telephone calls, or drill you about who called you, who wrote you a letter, or what you were talking about?
.70 Make you account for every minute you spend away from the house?
.65 Become jealous about your friends, family or pets?
.62 Ask for detailed reports of your hourly activities?
.61 Check up on you throughout the day? (calls you every 15 minutes, comes home early from work, has others tell him your whereabouts, etc.)
.57 Threaten to hurt a prized possession, pets, friends, or relatives if you don't comply with his wishes?
.48 Keep you up late yelling at you, either accusing you of having affairs or accusing you of other things?

Ignore
Internal Alpha Reliability = .80

.77 Make the TV, a magazine, the newspaper, or other people seem more important than you are?
.74 Ignore your need for assistance when you're sick, tired, or over-worked?
.71 Complain or ridicule you if you are upset or ask for emotional support?
.70 Ignore your suggestion to have sex or not do what excites or satisfies you?
.61 Ignore you when you begin a conversation?

Ridicule Traits
Internal Alpha Reliability = .79

.80 Ridicule the traits you admire or value most in yourself?
.66 Tell you that you are a horrible lover, worthless, or no good?
.54 Suggest you're crazy or stupid?
.50 Call you names with sexual connotations such as "slut" or "whore" or "cunt"?
.46 Make fun of your triumphs, discourage your plans, or minimize your successes?

Criticize Behavior
Internal Alpha Reliability = .75

.73 After you've cooked or cleaned, tell you it's not right and ask you to do it over again until he decides it's done right?
.61 Inspect your work and make overly critical comments?
.50 Request that everything be done in a precise way or it will be unacceptable to him?

Fear of Abuse
Internal Alpha Reliability = .84

Make you feel guilty or ashamed for something he demanded that you do?
Make you feel you as if you are "walking on egg shells" when you are around him?
How often:
Do you worry that what you do will make your partner angry?
Do you do things your partner wants you to do because you feel afraid?
Do you fear that your partner will hit you if you don't comply with his wishes?
Do you try to second-guess how your partner will act?

Index

Verbal aggression:
   control and, 155
   incidence of, 4
   impact of, generally, 154-155
   physical aggression and, 13-14
Victimization, women's response to,
   148. *See also* Strategic responses
Violence, *see specific types of abuse
   and aggression*
   defined, 120
   level of, 165
Vulnerability, 157

Ways of Coping Checklist-Revised
   (WCCL-R), 142, 144
Weapons, 180
Welfare reform, impact of, 119, 128
Well-being:
   marital, 162
   psychological, in women, 148, 157,
   168
Wife Abuse Inventory, 105, 121
Wiggins' Revised Interpersonal

Adjective Scale, 35
Withdrawal, emotional, 30, 169
Witnesses, in criminal cases, 185
Work/school interference:
   future research directions, 130
   measures, 124-125
   methodology, 122-124
Work/School Abuse Scale (W/SAS):
   description of, 124-125
   development of, 122
   factor structure, 130
   frequencies, 126
   Interference Tactics, 127-129
   limitations of, 130
   psychometric properties, 126
   purpose of, 131
   reliability of, 125, 127-128, 130
   Restraint Tactics, 127-129
   subscales, 128, 130
   text of, 133
   validity, 127-128, 130

Zeitgeist, 6

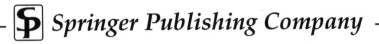
SP *Springer Publishing Company*

Ending Spouse / Partner Abuse
A Psychoeducational Approach for Individuals and Couples

Robert Geffner, PhD, with **Carol Mantooth,** MS

"By offering eclectic interventions together with a balanced, non-judgmental therapeutic stance, Ending Spouse/Partner Abuse *heralds the future of anti-violence counseling."*
—**Behavioral Science Book Service**

This clinician's manual and workbook contains a 26-session treatment plan to reduce wife/partner maltreatment. Geffner and Mantooth describe an abuse intervention model that incorporates various theories of psychotherapy. The techniques of this model have been implemented by abuse help centers for over a decade.

The authors include comprehensive weekly counseling sessions that address how to initiate the therapeutic relationship; communicate and express feelings; teach self-management and assertiveness techniques; discuss intimacy issues; and implement a relapse prevention program. Each session contains brief intervention regimens, handouts, and homework assignments. The flexible modification of materials in the manual benefit the trained clinician with specific client needs.

For therapists and counselors who treat domestic partner abuse. Workbook available in English and Spanish.

Partial Contents:
  I. Foundations and Brief Interventions • II. Communicating and Expressing Feelings • III. Self-Management and Assertiveness • IV. Intimacy Issues and Relapse Prevention Monthly Sessions

1999   400pp.   0-8261-1269-2   soft
1999   400pp.   0-8261-1289-7   soft
www.springerpub.com

536 Broadway, New York, NY 10012-3955 • (212) 431-4370 • Fax (212) 941-7842

Springer Publishing Company

Sexual Violence on Campus
Policies, Programs and Perspectives

Allen J. Ottens, PhD and **Kathy Hotelling,** PhD, ABPP, Editors

A somber reminder that sexual aggression, violence, and rape are chronic and serious problems on college campuses today, this volume proposes proactive steps for remedying the situation. It addresses the relationship of alcohol and rape; includes the latest information on club drugs and drug-facilitated rape; and explores the special issues around gay, lesbian and transgender violence. Chapters also address changing "the culture" found in and often fostered by fraternities and sororities as well as some athletic teams. It also contains constructive strategies for preventing sexual assault, managing anger, counseling survivor groups, and more. This book will arm counselors and administrators with the ammunition necessary to stop sexual assault on college campuses across the country.

Contents:

2000   328pp   0-8261-1374-5   hardcover

536 Broadway, New York, NY 10012 • **(212)431-4370** • **Fax: (212)941-7842**
Order Toll-Free: 1-877-687-7476 • *www.springerpub.com*